Food Security in a Global Economy

Food Security in a Global Economy

Veterinary Medicine and Public Health

Edited by
Gary Smith and Alan M. Kelly

PENN

University of Pennsylvania Press
Philadelphia

Published by
University of Pennsylvania Press
Philadelphia, Pennsylvania 19104-4112

Printed in the United States of America on acid-free paper

10 9 8 7 6 5 4 3 2 1

A Cataloging-in-Publication (CIP) record
is available from the Library of Congress.

ISBN 978-0-8122-2044-5

Contents

II. The Food Industry

III. Emerging Threats

IV. National and Global Responses

Foreword:
A Note on Martin Kaplan
Lord Soulsby of Swaffham Prior

It is especially appropriate that a volume dedicated to discussing veterinary public health in a global economy begin by highlighting a University of Pennsylvania Veterinary School alumnus whose career captures how veterinary medicine intersects with public health.

Martin Kaplan was born in Philadelphia on June 23, 1915, and died in Geneva, Switzerland, on October 16, 2004, at the age of 89. He received his professional education at Penn's School of Veterinary Medicine, graduating in 1940.

After a brief period in private practice in Philadelphia, he joined the United Nations Relief and Rehabilitation Administration (UNRRA), and on V-E Day—Victory in Europe Day, May 8, 1945—sailed to Greece, escorting six prize bulls donated by the Brethren Society of Pennsylvania for the purpose of restocking the decimated cattle population of Greece. He then joined the Food and Agriculture Organization (FAO) in Rome, where he performed similar work in various countries.

Martin Kaplan was a friend of Albert Einstein and on his return home was, at Einstein's behest, induced to become dean of the veterinary school of what is now Brandeis University. Through no fault of Kaplan's, the project fell through, and Einstein withdrew his support. Nevertheless, Einstein had a strong influence on him, encouraging him to take a stand against injustice and to reach across national barriers in search of peaceful solutions to the world's conflicts. This led him to join the Pugwash Conferences on Science and World Affairs later in his career.

In 1947 Kaplan rejoined the FAO and, while bound for an assignment in China, was asked to stop in Poland to organize a symposium. During the next few months the Chinese revolution moved toward its final stages, and he was forced to cancel his China plans. In 1949 he joined the evolving World Health Organization (WHO) in Geneva, to form a Veterinary Division. The following years were the most formative in Kaplan's veterinary career and were important to world veterinary public health. He created a highly effective Veterinary Division in WHO, recruiting distinguished veterinary scientists from around the world. He also pioneered investigations on influenza in birds and, together with Dr. Hilary Koprowski at the Wistar Institute, worked on a successful vaccine for rabies.

Kaplan's accomplishments in the Veterinary Division of WHO led him to become Director of Science and Technology in the Office of the Director General of WHO. He believed strongly that human health and animal health are closely associated and that neither can prosper effectively without the other, especially in the developing world. The premise of his 1971 essay, "Science and Social Values," is as valid today as it was then: "we are faced with war, poverty, increasing disorder and social alienation, distorted priorities, declining freedoms and individual powerlessness. These are products not of man's inherent evil but of the inexorable grinding of the national machines with their imperatives of growth, profit and glory."

In 1958 Kaplan joined the Pugwash Conferences on Science and World Affairs, a movement dedicated to bringing together scientists of the world in the interests of peace and in particular the control of weapons of mass destruction. In 1976 he retired from WHO and became Secretary General of the Pugwash Conferences; he devoted the next dozen years to that cause, work that led in 1995 to the awarding of the Nobel Peace Prize to the organization and its founder, Sir Joseph Rotblat.

Martin Kaplan, through his work in science, at WHO in veterinary medicine and public health, and finally in the Pugwash movement, was a man of giant intellect and global influence. He is an alumnus Penn's School of Veterinary Medicine remains proud of as it strives to perpetuate the outstanding work and ideals for which he stood.

Preface
Joan Hendricks

On November 8, 2006, Martin Kaplan's spirit animated the festive dinner initiating Penn Vet's first Conference on Veterinary Public Health in a Global Economy, which serves as the inspiration for this collection of essays. Martin's family and colleagues shared their memories and enthusiasms with many who hoped to be part of his legacy: veterinarians and scientists wishing to use the unique training and talents of the veterinary profession to change the world.

Martin Kaplan was born on June 23, 1915, and in his eighty-nine years he became arguably the world's most influential veterinarian, and certainly the most illustrious graduate of Penn's School of Veterinary Medicine. His career included leadership in world health organizations until 1976 and a major and instrumental role in the Pugwash movement, which was awarded the Nobel Peace Prize in 1995 for its work on the threat posed by weapons of mass destruction. At a time when veterinarians were commonly seen as more mechanics than scientists, how did Martin achieve global prominence?

One answer lies in his experience. He played a pivotal role in many of the international health initiatives of his time, as detailed in Lord Soulsby's foreword. While shaped by his times and experiences, Martin Kaplan's own character was clearly central to his influence. He was a charismatic, visionary, and inspired man. At that dinner, as we shared memories and photographs of Martin and other people of towering stature, including many of the 2006 conference participants, the strength and warmth of this remarkable veterinarian and political activist enlivened us. The meeting that followed carried forward the spirit of cohesiveness and resolve that Martin embodied in his lifetime to a new generation of veterinary scientists. The conference was truly one of enlightened thought, with lively and excited thinking that infused the entire meeting— during presentations, discussion, and perhaps most dynamically in the exchanges in the hallways and lobbies. Many presenters knew Martin personally, but by the end of the conference we all felt we had met him and were committed to carrying on his spirit by acting on our training and talents and energies to make the biggest possible impact on the quality of life for animals and society together, globally. We can only hope that we will succeed.

I wish to thank Martin's family and friends who supported and attended the conference, Alan Kelly for his inspirational leadership in organizing the first of what we expect to be a series of conferences, and Martin himself for being such a remarkable person. We look forward to producing new programs and training new Penn Vet graduates to make him and his family proud—and, most important, to change the world.

Introduction
Setting the Scene
Alan M. Kelly

At the end of the nineteenth century, the health and productivity of the livestock and poultry industries and the safety of foods of animal origin in the United States were severely compromised by infectious diseases. Bovine tuberculosis was widespread and a significant food safety hazard, with large numbers of human TB cases coming from contaminated milk. Texas fever, foot-and-mouth disease, brucellosis, glanders, trichinosis, and fowl plague (avian influenza) were among other infections that challenged both animal and human health. In 1884 the U.S. government formed the Bureau of Animal Industries with the charge of inventing and executing programs in veterinary public health. Led by Daniel Salmon, the Bureau included a brilliant group of public health veterinarians who uncovered the tick-borne cause of Texas fever while discovering the involvement of arthropods in the transmission of infectious agents. The Bureau's contributions to public health were immense, especially during the first half of the twentieth century, as it designed ways of eradicating many infections, including bovine TB, and wrote legislation to support the control strategies. Now, 125 years later, though the risks remain, losses from infectious diseases in the American livestock and poultry industries are greatly reduced, and the U.S. food supply is proclaimed to be the safest in the world.

In the countries of the developing world, infectious diseases of animals and humans are still prevalent and pose serious threats to a globalized society, in which economies and ways of life are increasingly interconnected. Although the nineteenth century looks like the distant past from a twenty-first-century perspective, the risks to American consumers are as urgent as those that confronted the Bureau of Animal Industries in 1884. The ongoing H5N1 avian influenza epidemic, for example, has shown that despite enormous advances in technology, Americans and their farm animals are as vulnerable to epidemics of viral infectious disease today as they were 125 years ago. The veterinary profession's established responsibility is to protect the health of the nation's livestock and poultry populations and the safety of the food supply. Veterinarians must now learn to accomplish this in the new paradigm of global health, because the health status of animals in one nation is directly linked to the health status of animal populations throughout the world. But the problems and their solutions are immensely complex and difficult, and extend well beyond the challenges of controlling infectious diseases. At the same time, the profession must recognize that public health is a political pursuit and that veterinary medicine presently has no formidable lobby.

The issues primarily concern the developing world, where population growth is estimated to increase by some 50 percent over the next forty years and where social structures are changing radically. In large numbers, people are migrating far from their traditional farming communities to mushrooming cities that lack urban infrastructure, enforcement of health and waste disposal statutes, and effective veterinary public health services. Compounding the problem is the escalating demand for foods of animal origin and proliferating American-style supermarkets and fast food chains selling hamburgers, hot dogs, and fried chicken. These markets are supplied by livestock and poultry industries that have been revolutionized to intensive, Westernized systems. Owing to the poor quality of roads and a dearth of cold chain facilities to control temperatures, intensive animal operations are commonly located in peri-urban areas. Though some are well managed, others lack adequate biosecurity and expose huge numbers of animals to infectious agents, especially those coming from wildlife. They also produce vast quantities of manure that is discharged into streams and rivers, leading to serious environmental damage. In view of all this, those involved in the food industry, and especially veterinarians, need to ask themselves the question, "Is it possible to feed a burgeoning world population while respecting the welfare of livestock and poultry, containing the spread of disease, and managing Earth's natural resources?" These are issues of immense social concern and form the central challenge for veterinary medicine in the twenty-first century.

A Road Map

The contributors to this volume come from differing disciplines, but they are all concerned about the continued health of our fragile planet.

The book opens with a discussion by Gregg BeVier on the future of global agriculture and the intrinsic veterinary partnership. After surveying the landscape, BeVier finishes with the loaded question, "Are veterinarians prepared to invent their future?"

In Chapter 2, Stephen Kobrin explores globalization, what causes it, and how it will end. He raises a question not frequently asked: "Is it here to stay?" He goes on to point out that if globalization is here to stay, the development of an effective multilateral system of governance will not be an easy or rapid process. This critical theme of global agreements on food production, disease control, and health echoes throughout the book.

Cornelis de Haan and Henning Steinfeld (Chapter 3) follow Kobrin with discussions on the impact of globalization on society, hunger, the risks to human, animal, and environmental health associated with the "livestock revolution," and the changing landscape of veterinary public health in the globalized twenty-first century. De Haan and Steinfeld make the point that veterinarians will need to be trained to address the global challenges associated with population growth and increased food animal production in the developing world.

Globalization came about as a result of advances in technology, particularly in transportation and digital communication. Advances in technology must be the solution to many of the challenges facing the global food industry today. In Chapter 4, David Galligan and Edward Kanara give the example of the remarkable increases in milk production in America's dairy herds over the past fifty years. They argue that the same method must be applied around the world to meet demand. Production efficiency is key: although it may not be immediately obvious, production efficiency is directly linked to protecting the environment and biodiversity. Moreover, reducing total feed intake per unit of production reduces the manure load and the risk of pollution of precious water resources. To achieve high yields of milk, pork, or poultry while at the same time ensuring biosecurity inescapably means intensive systems of production. These systems admittedly come with their own set of risks but seem inevitable in Southeast Asia, where human populations are burgeoning and there is insufficient land to do otherwise.

A sense of the risks associated with livestock production is outlined in Chapter 5 by Paul B. Thompson. He compares the short supply chain that marked much of nineteenth-century America's food production, with livestock locally raised and butchered, to the long supply chain in twenty-first-century America, with distance and multiple supply and distribution points the dominant model. Gary Smith, in Chapter 6, also looks back to a time when animals played central economic and military roles, and how those roles were endangered by "animal plagues" that could play havoc on the security of the state. Smith also shows how the global spread of animal plagues was as much a concern then as it is today.

Trade is at the core of globalization, promoting economic growth and in turn alleviating poverty and hunger. In agriculture, globalization has also promoted consolidation, vertical integration, and business growth. Part II opens with an admirable discussion by

David Harlan and Candace Jacobs on the global food industry. Wal-Mart, Tyson, ConAgra, Cargill, and H-E-B Foods have grown to be international food companies of such size that they strongly influence world markets, a fact that unsettles many governments. Harlan and Jacobs point out that the greatest challenge for international companies trading in meat is disease. Failure to implement global, science-based trade standards has a huge impact on the ability of food corporations to use risk management strategies to anticipate and manage disease. It is in the food corporations' best interest to promote public-private partnerships in which all stakeholders share the risk and responsibility as they endeavor to harmonize trading policies. Jacobs echoes this by observing that supermarkets dominate the way food is handled globally, and American-style supermarkets are increasingly the standard for food safety, animal welfare, and environmental protection around the world.

The global food industry has had to deal with growing demand for meat products as consumers have grown more affluent. In some parts of the world, however, the demand, driven by rising incomes, is for seafood. Meeting this demand is the focus of Richard Langan's chapter on aquaculture. Langan notes that, while aquaculture production has increased nearly 10 percent annually since 1980, it has not kept up with demand. He sketches a potential solution that makes use of open ocean "fish farming" that is environmentally sustainable and technologically feasible.

The growth in demand for livestock products has meant more intense livestock production, which has also led to an increase in antibiotics. The impact of this growing use of antibiotics is the subject of Chapter 9, by Shelley Rankin, who explores the dimensions of the problem and the international response.

Part III addresses specific emerging threats to humans from animals. In Chapter 10, Ilaria Capua, D. J. Alexander, Bruce Rideout, and Martin Vincent provide an outstanding discussion of the current situation regarding the highly pathogenic H5N1 avian influenza virus. They point to the complexity of developing global accords for the control of new and emerging infectious diseases in animals and humans. Most of these infections originate in wildlife, where, it is now realized, they are naturally confined within ecological niches defined by their host species. When humans or domestic animals encroach on these niches they create new opportunities for cross-species transmission of disease. For example, the current global epidemic of avian influenza probably originated in rice paddies of Southeast Asia that had been wetland sanctuaries. Subsequent viral transmission to backyard poultry permitted mutation to the highly pathogenic H5N1 variant, which then spread rapidly through an industry experiencing years of unregulated growth. H5N1 also spread from poultry back to wild birds, where it killed many and, ominously, may have become endemic in some wild bird populations. As the authors discuss, this is an obvious concern that requires implementation of a global system of surveillance, reporting, and containment and is an issue that policy makers must immediately address.

Chapters 11 and 12 extend this theme. Bruno Chomel presents a detailed review of the remarkably wide-ranging ways in which zoonoses have been transmitted from wildlife to domestic animals and humans during the past decade. No one situation is the same as the next. Darin Carroll focuses on one good example, the transmission of monkeypox to the United States in 2003. Monkeypox is endemic to the Congo Basin; it was transmitted to the United States in an airborne shipment of small rodents from Ghana. When exposed to monkeypox, prairie dogs, lacking natural immunity, became severely affected and subsequently transmitted the disease to humans. As Carroll points out, the introduction of monkeypox into the United States illustrates how easily globalization can cause a breach in the ecological compartmentalization that tends to keep us safe.

Chapter 13, by Charles Rupprecht, Lin-Fa Wang, and Leslie Real, deals with rabies, severe acute respiratory syndrome (SARS), and Ebola virus disease (hemorrhagic fever), all of which are considered to be bat zoonoses. Rabies is the most widespread, affecting all mammals and killing humans by the thousands every year despite persistent efforts at control. Although rabies is usually identified with dogs, raccoons, and foxes, this chapter reveals that the virus originated in bats, having persisted in insectivorous bats for thousands of years before spilling over into terrestrial mammals. The authors propose that bats, ubiquitous flying mammals, spread the virus around the world. Furthermore, they project that no nation can claim to be free of rabies based on control programs that are limited to terrestrial mammals.

Bats are also the reservoir host of the virus that causes SARS, the infection that suddenly spilled over into palm civets and humans in 2003, causing high rates of mortality and huge financial losses as it spread around the world. The authors describe work that identified horseshoe bats as the reservoir host of the SARS virus and opened the way for rapidly controlling the epidemic. The reservoir host of Ebola virus is also suspected to be bats, probably fruit bats, though conclusive evidence of this is still lacking. The chapter explores the spread of Ebola Zaire, the most deadly species of Ebola virus, among gorillas and humans in Gabon and Zaire starting in 1976. In contrast to rabies, the spillover of Ebola infection to gorillas is a recent event that has developed into an ongoing epidemic, spreading from gorilla to gorilla and decimating their population. Human infections appear to be a side event from this epidemic, resulting from exposure to contaminated bushmeat. The chapter highlights the present dearth of understanding of zoonotic diseases of wildlife. The reservoir host of Ebola virus must be resolved as one of many urgent questions requiring investment in research on bats and other hard to study animals.

The final section of the book considers current national and global responses. The contribution by François-Xavier Meslin and Corrie Brown focuses on early detection of new disease outbreaks, especially of zoonotic disease, and the development of techniques to predict when these emergencies may develop. An important development Meslin and Brown report is the landmark agreement among the World Organization for Animal Health (known by its French abbreviation, OIE), the World Health Organization (WHO), and the Food and Agriculture Organization (FAO) to integrate the early warning, alert, and response systems each organization has developed independently into one platform for enhanced warning and response to zoonotic disease outbreaks. This is an important first step toward a comprehensive global program that links veterinary and human public health services together. But, as the authors point out, there is the potential to do much more. They present a vision of the high-tech public health services of the twenty-first century that integrate open source computerized data gathering with mathematical models predicting when and where new disease outbreaks may occur, digital technologies that transmit high-quality images from field operations, and satellite remote sensing of environmental conditions that favor disease outbreaks, especially as the result of global warming.

Hugh Mainzer, in a spirited conclusion to the book, defines veterinary public health in the widest possible context and urges the profession to break out of the traditional realms of zoonoses and food safety. Mainzer's challenge echoes the question posed by BeVier in Chapter 1: "Are veterinarians prepared to invent their future?" The issues Mainzer raises are crucial not only to the threat of epidemics from zoonotic diseases but also to global hunger, food security, and the management of Earth's precious resources. The solution to these problems requires leadership from veterinarians working in collaboration with scientists from many different disciplines. It also requires the development of international agreements on trade, food safety, carbon credit trading, disease surveillance and control, wildlife habitats, and environmental protection. To prepare for this complex paradigm of global public health, veterinary schools must enlarge the window through which their students view the world. Producing sufficient food to sustain the world's burgeoning population without destroying the environment is the greatest public health challenge of the twenty-first century. Veterinary medicine has a professional and ethical responsibility to be centrally involved in this quest.

Part I
The Changing Landscape for Veterinary Public Health

Chapter 1
What Will the Future Bring, and How Can We Prepare for It?

Gregg W. BeVier

An Overview of Global Population and Agriculture

What would you attempt to do if you knew you would not fail? This is a challenge I would like veterinarians to consider. Would you parachute from an airplane, quit your job, or take business from a competitor? My hope is that this introductory chapter will provide insight into future opportunities for the veterinary profession, some specific recommendations on tools to consider, and the motivation to act—now.

My topic is the prediction of and preparation for the future, but what future and whose future? Much has been written about animal health, consumer trends, and livestock production issues such as welfare, residues, food safety, environmental safety, and genetic modification, and these topics will continue to challenge our industry. For now, however, I would like to step back for a moment and reflect on the future of global agriculture and the intrinsic veterinary partnership. Are we positioning ourselves for our future in global agriculture and food systems? My premise is that the personal investment and effort needed are equally important to the technical challenges we face.

The purpose of global agriculture is to feed the world. The world population has a growth rate of about 1.2 percent per year.[1] When viewed over time, the past 200 years and the next 100 years represent a period of exponential population growth.[2] Six times as many people are alive today as were alive at the start of the Industrial Revolution, thirteen times more than when Columbus set sail, and twenty times more than during the Roman Empire.[3] There is a major demographic fault line between the pace of growth in developing and industrialized nations. Essentially 99 percent of all future population increase will take place in poor countries, while the population in the rich nations is static or declining (except in the United States).[4] The current world population is 6.4 billion and is expected to reach 9.4 billion people by 2050.[5] The global maximum for planet Earth has been estimated at 10 to 14 billion people. India is expected to supplant China as the most populous nation by 2050.[6]

Another demographic factor of interest is the shift toward urbanization, where "urban" denotes towns of more than 2,000 residents. In 1970, about two-thirds of the world lived in rural areas. By 2030, about two-thirds will be living in urban areas. The regions of the world differ greatly in their rate of urbanization: the less-developed countries are urbanizing at rapid rates. The catalyst for this shift toward urban growth is economic development. Despite predicted economic growth, more than 50 percent of the global population live on less than $2 per day, and 98 percent of the world's population live on less than $10,000 (purchasing power parity) per year. Roughly three to four billion people do not consume much meat because they cannot afford it. As income in developing countries rises, there will be a substantial increase in the demand for commodity crops, especially for animal feed use. India and China are likely to be the key drivers for additional demand of agricultural commodities.[7] As per capita incomes rise, people eat more (calories) and differently (more vegetable oils, meat, sugar, and wheat). This reflects the preferences of consumers whose rising incomes allow them to purchase more expensive and more highly valued foods.[7] There is a downside to urbanization. Today, 220 million people lack access to clean water, 420 million people do not have access to latrines, and 20 to 50 percent of municipal waste goes uncollected in developing world cities.[8]

Natural Resource Supply

Will there be enough food to supply all the people? The answer is yes: we have an abundance of food. The world food supplies have more than doubled in the past three decades, the quality of most diets has improved, and the real cost of food has declined.[8] The world produces enough grain each year to provide every human being on the planet with 3,500 calories per day.[9] That is enough for most of us to get fat if we could manage an all-grain diet. If one were to include all food—vegetables, fruits, meat, fish—produced each year, each person could be provided with about 4.3 lb of food a day (2.3 lb grain, beans, and nuts; 1 lb fruit and vegetables; 1 lb meat, milk, and eggs).[9] If the world's farmers could achieve the average yield of U.S. corn growers, a world of 10 billion people would need half of today's cropland while consuming today's American calories.[8] If the world's farmers could add 1.5 percent to their output each year, 10 billion people could eat an American-style diet (not that I suggest this) and still spare about 25 percent of available cropland.[8] As a side note, the U.S. Department of Agriculture (USDA) estimates that between production and end use, more than 25 percent of the food produced in the United States goes to waste. This equates to about 1 lb per person per day of wasted food.[10] Nevertheless, 800 million people in developing countries still suffer from chronic undernutrition, hunger, and food insecurity.[7] A study by the International Food Policy Research Institute reviewed trends in urban poverty and malnutrition in fourteen developing countries. In the majority of countries, the number of underweight children is rising faster in urban areas than in rural areas.[7] Undernutrition in childhood may lead to chronic health problems in adulthood. More than 40 percent of urban residents in developing countries live in slums. In many developing countries, the urban poor spend 60 percent of their total expenditures on food (compared to 11 percent in the United States). Poor people often buy more than half their meals from street food vendors, typically foods with high fat content and of questionable safety. Twelve million children die each year from hunger and hunger-related diseases. This is equivalent to the number of people killed instantly by a Hiroshima bomb every three days.[7] It should be noted that 78 percent of all malnourished children under five years of age in the developing world live in countries with food surpluses.[9]

What about our dry land resource? Is global agriculture managing this resource properly? The Earth's mass is occupied 70 percent by water and 30 percent by dry land. Of the dry land mass, 70 percent is used for agriculture. At current rates of destruction, the rain forests will be gone by 2031. Rain forests cover 7 percent of the planet yet are home to 50 percent of the world's species of plants and animals. The rain forests are important to life on Earth for other reasons: they are literally the lungs of the world because of their carbon dioxide consumption and oxygen production.[9] As livestock agriculture expands to meet future demand, we must carefully consider the environmental impacts of converting large tracts of forested land to the monoculture of animal feed crops. It has been estimated that the land deforested in Brazil between 2000 and 2006 was equivalent to an area larger than Greece (about 150,000 square kilometers).

The story of water follows that of food: generally sufficient global supplies marred by regional shortages. If the world's water could fit in a bathtub, the portion of it that could be used in a sustainable manner in any given year would almost fill a teaspoon.[8] Water scarcity will constrain agriculture primarily because high-yield crops require more water.[8] Conservation efforts can work, and greater efforts could be made. Between 1980 and 1895, the United States reduced water consumption by 10 percent, even as its population grew by 16 percent.[8]

Poverty, not an inadequate food supply, is the root cause of hunger. It has been said, "A poor person has many problems, but a hungry person has one problem." Human poverty is a direct result of government policy, which in the near term is unlikely to change enough to have a significant impact on hunger. Because of this political inertia, we must be able to triple the productivity of the world's agriculture over the next fifty years to meet the demands of a larger, more affluent, and aging (Western) world population.[8] We do not have three Earths to use as a resource.

Livestock Productivity, with Specific Reference to Pork

Let's examine why we need to consider tripling the pork supply by 2050 from current supplies. As previously mentioned, the global population is currently 6.4 billion. The global pork supply for the population is 93.5 billion metric tons. If we assume that the global sow inventory is 70 million sows that produce an average of thirteen pigs per sow per year, then we can begin to estimate the sow productivity required to satisfy the forecasted increase in population. There are three different growth scenarios for pork supply and the required pigs per sow per year (p/s/y) over the next forty-five years (assuming a constant sow base and no change in demand for pork). The first scenario is for the pork supply to match or be consistent with the forecasted population growth. In this scenario, we will need to attain a global average of 19.6 p/s/y by 2050. The second scenario utilizes an annual growth rate of 2.7 percent until the year 2050. This compound annual growth rate was selected because it is the same as that of a recent five-year period (2000–2005). Assuming no change in sow herd size or consumer demand, the global sow productivity would need to achieve 43.1 p/s/y by 2050. The third scenario uses a compound annual growth of 1.35 percent, or half of that seen in the period 2000–2005. With similar assumptions, by 2050 we would need to average 23.8 p/s/y globally. The total supply of pork relative to the human population is an important starting point for gauging world food needs over the coming decades.

The next critical issue pertains to the regional location where the pork is produced relative to the human population. We have enough food; it is just not where it needs to be at the right price. Table 1 depicts the forecasted change in the human population between 2005 and 2050 in three regions of the world. As Europe's percentage of the global population declines, will there be continued growth of pig meat production in this area? In regard to AASV membership, 83 percent of the current members ($n = 1,266$) reside in the Americas, an area representing 14 percent of the population and 17 percent of the global pig meat supply. If AASV membership growth is proportional to population growth, we should have 1,859 members by 2050.

Especially in developed nations, there will be an increase in public awareness regarding the health and nutrition of livestock and humans that will drive important changes in the food system. People are demanding more information about the food they consume. Traceability of all the food we consume will become commonplace. Customized, multiple product channels from farm to shelf will continue to grow, especially in the developed countries. Underdeveloped countries have specialized needs that the food industry has not begun to address. There are three key principles, referred to as the three A's, which identify how poor people make choices.[11] First is affordability. The increasing number of products sold in the simple-serve formats where people can spend pennies to purchase "one dose" of something is an example of affordability. Second is access to the product: poor people must work all day long and cannot travel all night to reach a store. The third principle is availability and distribution. This factor takes into account the variability of cash flow for the poor and their desire to purchase things when they have cash and their inability to purchase without cash (having no access to credit).

Sustainable systems that consider the environment, food safety, animal welfare, and natural resources will become standard. The veterinarian has an opportunity to be a key participant in driving

TABLE 1   Regional Differences in Human Population and Pork
Production (2005)

Region	% Human Population 2005	% Human Population 2050	% Pig Meat Production, 2005 (93.5 BMT)	% AASV Members (n = 226)
Asia	60	57	55	83
Europe	11	9	22	13
Americas	14	13	17	4
Rest of world	15	23	6	<1

Human population = 6.464 billion (2005), estimated 9.06 billion (2050).

Source: United Nations, Department of Economic and Social Affairs, Population Division, 2005 (www.un.org/esa).

these important changes and in "writing the food prescription" for the future health and welfare of livestock and humanity. I believe that as veterinarians, it is our mandate to ensure the food prescription for mankind.

Agribusiness Consolidation: A Swine Industry Example

Consolidation and globalization in agriculture will continue over the next decade. As a result of these trends, vertical integration of the food chain is expected to increase, as is the use of monocultures in crop and livestock production on larger farms. The poultry industry has established the model for livestock integration and expansion, and large pork integrators have essentially used the same plan of attack. This plan rests on four pillars. The first pillar is establishment of a large base of livestock supply by geographic expansion. Size will foster economies of scale, and globalization of the supply will be an important predecessor to long-term consumer distribution. Having a supply base in key markets mitigates the impact of non-tariff trade barriers and supply interruptions caused by global events. The second pillar is optimization of the vertically integrated model. With a large, consistent, high-quality raw material supply, the integrated model can optimize supply and demand dynamics. Long "run times" can be staged, and reducing switching costs by using consistent raw materials provides cost advantages with scale. Additionally, when compared with the nonintegrated model, the vertically integrated model should allow more consistent earnings to be achieved by having the live hog and the processed pork within the same entity. A consistent earnings profile is highly valued by the financial markets. The third pillar is maximizing the value from further processing. The balance sheet of an integrated operation generally shows that the bulk of capital investment is on the livestock side of the business, not the processing side. The incremental investment for processing and further processing of convenience foods is small in comparison. In addition, the processed products yield higher levels of profitability per pound when compared with fresh pork. It has been estimated that traditional processed pork (bacon) yields three to five cents more per pound in pretax profit than fresh pork. It has also been estimated that further processed pork (convenience foods and fully cooked products) yields eight to ten cents more per pound than fresh pork. Why should a nonintegrated investor take all the production risk and capital risk while forgoing the price premium from further processed products? The fourth pillar is application, over the long term, of a similar integrated model to other meats, including beef, chicken, turkey, and seafood, to address the global food supply challenge. With this pillar complete, the integrated livestock producer becomes a food producer capable of offering a "meat case" to the global consumer.

Consolidation in the global food industry and the increasing market power of large food retailers (such as Wal-Mart) will strengthen the domestic and worldwide influence of a few marketing decisions, such as the decision to introduce genetically modified organisms. Some people refer to this dominance of the world's food supply by a few large corporations as "food dictatorship," pointing to the lack of freedom of choice resulting from corporate control and consumer dependency.[12] Many governments, on the other hand, see food sovereignty as an issue of national security. Terrorism events help reinforce the notion that greater oversight and control of a nation's food supply is vital to national security. I do not believe consolidation is something we should fear. We need to understand the motives and be prepared to participate actively so that systems are established in a manner consistent with the food prescription we will help to write.

The Green Revolution and the Livestock Revolution

To get a better feel for the future opportunity for livestock, it is useful to compare the factors involved in the Green Revolution with those affecting how the livestock sector may grow. The Green Revolution occurred in the 1980s in developed countries with crops (corn, beans, wheat, cotton). Stepwise changes in the technology of seeds (genetic modification) and fertilizer occurred that improved crop yields and drove a supply-side revolution. As happens with most revolutions, there was considerable adverse reaction to the green revolution in key markets. This negative public reaction illustrates the concept of food dictatorship felt by the consumer.

The story is different for the livestock sector. Dairy and poultry producers in developed countries initially led the way, introducing technological advances in livestock production. Fortunately, genetic modification was not the key technology utilized initially to foster improvements in livestock productivity. The biggest difference from the crop revolution is that the livestock revolution is expected to be demand driven in the future by the less-developed countries. Known technology, rather than genetically modified technology, will be applied in sustainable systems.

Some key characteristics are emerging in association with the future of livestock production. Global increases in both the production and the consumption of livestock products are unavoidable. Most of the increases in both production and consumption will occur in the less-developed countries. Consumption trends point to the substitution of meat and milk for grain in the diet of humans. This substitution will drive up the demand for grain production for livestock feed. Livestock production will become more technical, intensive, specialized, and integrated. This system will put more stress on the land and the environment. A rapid rate of technical change throughout the entire food chain system will be needed to meet these developments in a sustainable manner. In essence, we have a global market demand that is waiting for meat to be supplied at the right place, time, quality, and price. I believe this is an opportunity of a lifetime.

Livestock Production: Consolidation, Integration, Globalization

Profound spatial changes in the relationship of plants, animals, and humans have occurred over the past millennium; forthcoming changes will be much more rapid. A major change, one evident today, is the concentration of agriculture ownership and control in the hands of transnational corporations. In countries such as Chile, the United States, Brazil, Canada, Spain, and Mexico, the top ten pork producers account for 20 to 30 percent of the national sow herd (with the noteworthy exception of Chile, where the top ten producers own 90 percent of the sows). The same trend exists for the processing segment. In Denmark, Chile, Canada, Mexico, the United States, Germany, and Spain, three to five pork processors maintain a market share of 18 to 95 percent. Five U.S. chicken processors together have about a 60 percent market share, and five U.S. beef processors have a 90 percent market share. Supplier and retailer concentration is likewise occurring. The top three animal genetic suppliers for avian, bovine, and porcine species have leading market shares of the global genetic market. The top three animal health companies have 50 percent of the global animal health market. From a retail perspective, the top fifteen food retailers have a 30 percent market share of the food sold at retail, a $2 trillion global market.[13]

We are in the middle of a consolidation period where new connections are being established that will greatly affect the supply, cost, and quality of the food we eat. This trend will continue for decades to come, but, "as the big get bigger," we will once again see inefficiencies, because no single monolithic organization can do it all. There will be opportunities for outsourcing activities to specialized niche players who can add unique value. It will be up to us to invent the new value opportunities.

Livestock Productivity and Enterprise Costs

The adage "It's all about the cost of production" is a pervasive concept in global agriculture production, and in high-throughput manufacturing businesses in general. A driving economic force is the balance between economies and diseconomies of scale. A business tries to achieve the point of maximum efficiency. Another important aspect for cost and output relates to capital and labor. Capital substitution for labor will continue to be the key investment priority for livestock production and the entire food chain in the future, to achieve improved levels of output at the right cost. As labor costs and availability (willingness) continue to challenge our production systems, automation will more frequently replace manual labor on the farm. These investments are required to meet the demand for meat in the future. If livestock production is viewed as a commodity, then it is reasonable to expect an enormous effort to improve unit costs. But this perspective has turned production agriculture into a cost center for the entire food supply chain. In essence, the profit margins move along the chain toward the retailer while the producer accepts lower margins and hopefully a lower risk profile. Our singular focus on cost has put the producer in this position, and marketing programs for meat will not mitigate the high cost of operations. Perhaps if we could achieve a better balance between our costs and satisfying the needs of the consumer, we could recapture some of this lost margin in the future.

The pervasive low-cost attitude regarding production has inspired all of us to find ways to increase biological productivity metrics. Since all costs are variable in the long run, every cent of cost should be challenged. The poultry firms have made a science of this practice. Improved nutrition, housing, genetics, health, and management have been the key tools, and the poultry industry has done an exceptional job of mastering the use of these tools. There have been impressive gains in broiler performance over the past eighty years: in 1925 it took 112 days to get a broiler to a market weight of 2.5 lb, whereas in 2005 it took 44 days to get a broiler to a market weight of 5.25 lb. We should focus on operational excellence because even today in the United States a large gap exists between the performance of the average producer and that of the top 10 percent. For example, in the U.S. swine industry, the difference in the number of pigs weaned per sow per year between the top 10 percent and the bottom 10 percent of farms is about six pigs per sow per year. If the bottom 10 percent of farms could produce at the rate of the top 10 percent, we could increase the national supply of pigs by more than 3.5 percent. This is where the real opportunities exist for the next decade in global production agriculture. To initiate operational excellence will require an unprecedented focus at the point of production on livestock health, not disease.

The Nature of Health

The health and well-being of livestock is an emotional topic, and different animal industries take different approaches. Swine producers have gone to great lengths to learn how to live with animal diseases. Poultry producers have gone to similar lengths to prevent them. There are reasons for the approach taken by the swine industry; however, once these reasons become acceptable, a line is crossed that is difficult to erase.

Many variables in agriculture can be controlled or locked in. Grain can be forward purchased, utility services can be priced with noninterruption guarantees, breeding stock and packer agreements are multiyear in scope. But there are also variables that cannot be so easily dealt with. Weather and disease outbreaks cannot be easily controlled and do dramatically affect our food systems. Foot-and-mouth disease, BSE, blue tongue, and avian influenza are but a few animal disease examples of recent history. Weather forecasters have gone to great lengths to model weather patterns and forecast the future. They are not always right, and we do not always listen to their input. We must improve our ability to predict when "conditions are favorable" to cause an interruption in health status. Once outbreaks occur, we need better models and intervention protocol (such as vaccines) to diminish the economic impact of the disease. We also need to provide advice on long-term solutions for disease elimination. The poultry industry has an arsenal of effective vaccines, mostly delivered in ovo so that when the chick hatches it never needs to be touched and is protected during the growth phase. This industry has also utilized premise depopulation as an effective method to break the disease cycle and return to high levels of health. Is it too radical to believe that someday we could have piglets immunized at parturition against all the pathogens they may encounter? That someday we could find a cost-effective way to depopulate, on a regional basis, to stop the spread of disease? The health status of livestock is our Achilles' heel, not our future profit center. Diagnosis and treatment are rearview mirror actions. Prevention is the name of the game.

Livestock Veterinarians: Supply and Demand

Over the past twenty years, major changes have occurred in the veterinary workforce in the United States. More than 80 percent of veterinary schools have female students enrolled, and more than 80 percent of graduates enter companion animal practice on graduation. Numerous reports have forecasted a shortage of food animal practitioners in the near future. The supply of food animal veterinarians will begin to increase only when new career opportunities in this area develop. It is up to us to invent these opportunities.

We do have some key tools at our disposal. Innovation is one of these. Innovation occurs by change and transformation. It involves new methods, creativity, ingenuity, and a dose of inspiration. Earlier I noted that technology and capital are required to drive future livestock supplies. An investment in personal development is just as important. When applied correctly, it can transform the way we work and the way people see our work. Let me suggest that further competencies for veterinarians are needed in business, finance, economics, supply chain, marketing, sales, leadership, general management, strategy, business development, human resources, and training.

A New Model for Veterinarians

To craft a new value curve with a better understanding of business, we should first challenge the basic business model food animal veterinarians utilize and ask four key questions.[14] First, "Which elements of the services provided by veterinarians does the industry take for granted and could be eliminated?" Income from the sales of drugs might be an example. The next question to ask is "Which elements of the services provided by veterinarians could be lowered well below the industry's current standard?" Here we might consider reducing the client's perception of the veterinarian as a doctor or technician. The third question is, "Which elements of the services provided by veterinarians could be elevated above the norm for the industry?" An example here might be charging more per hour or day, repositioning the provider as a business person with technical training, aligning compensation with farm performance, or engaging in a higher level of production management, including animal welfare, food safety, and consumer preferences. And fourth, "What new veterinary services could be created that have not been offered previously?" Examples of such services include ensuring food safety, animal welfare, and verification.

There are three characteristics of a good strategy for the new business model. The first characteristic is focus. The focus should be on the consumer, and on aligning all activities on the production chain toward fulfilling unmet consumer needs. I believe one of these needs will pertain to the food prescription. The second characteristic is divergence. Divergence refers to looking at all possible alternatives, not simply benchmarking competitors or other food animal veterinarians. Our ability to capture all aspects of the production chain would be an example of divergence. If done correctly, new ways to differentiate will become apparent. The third characteristic of a good strategy is to reconstruct the market boundaries and not be confined to a review of typical competitors. For example, if veterinarians are involved in "writing the food prescription," the competitors might be food retailers and pharmacists and not other veterinary practices.

Conclusion

Poverty, not inability to produce food, causes hunger. More food will be needed over the next forty years to meet the needs of a growing population. Some believe the amount of food needed could be three times the supply available today. Veterinarians have a key role to play in advancing and ensuring the food supply and food prescription for humans. We should learn from the Green Revolution and step up to the meat supply challenge for underdeveloped countries.

There are two key ways to strengthen our future. First is innovation via role expansion fostered by education and experience. The second way is by measuring our contribution. Veterinarians and other health professionals have not recorded metrics that demonstrate the value of their contributions. In the future, this will become a requirement for our sustainable input.

We could more than triple the size of this organization in ten years and add $390 million of veterinary income if we acted today. The food chain needs us, but I often wonder if we as a group envision this huge responsibility and opportunity. The 50 percent of the world's population living on less than $2 per day will eat more meat in the future if it is available at the right price. It is our challenge to help meet this need. It is time for veterinarians to stretch their thinking and take an adventurous look into the future of prescription food and satisfying human hunger on a global basis. Over three billion consumers in underdeveloped countries represent a key driver for meat demand. Technology will certainly play a role in improving output, but this should not be our only focus. The tools of personal innovation and measurement are waiting to be picked up and utilized. What would you attempt to do if you knew you would not fail? Are veterinarians prepared to invent their future?

References

1. Earth Policy Institute (2005), Eco-Economy Indicators: 2004 Population Growth, www.earth-policy.org.
2. UN Economic and Social Development Section, Population Division (1998), World Population Projection to 2150, Population Reference Bureau 2005, www.prb.org.
3. Population Awareness/Scripps Howard News Service (2005).
4. Population Reference Bureau (2005), 2004 World Population Data Sheet, www.prb.org.
5. U.S. Census Bureau (2005), *Global Population Profile: 2004* (New York: U.S. Census Bureau, Population Division).
6. Population Reference Bureau (2005), The World's Ten Largest Countries, www.prb.org.com.
7. Food and Agriculture Organization (2005), The State of Food Insecurity in the World, 2004, International Food Policy Research Institute Report, www.fao.org.
8. M. Mazarr (1999), *Global Trends 2005: An Owner's Manual for the Next Decade*, Center for Strategic and International Studies (New York: St. Martin's Press).
9. F. M. Lappe, J. Collins, and P. Rosset (1998), *World Hunger: Twelve Myths*, 2nd ed., Institute for Food and Development Policy (New York: Grove Press).
10. T. Dyson (2001), *Population and Food: Global Trends and Future Prospects* (London: Routledge).
11. C. K. Prahalad (2005), *The Fortune at the Bottom of the Pyramid* (Upper Saddle River, N.J.: Wharton School Publishing), 5.
12. V. Shiva (2003), "Food Democracy v. Food Dictatorship," presented at Future of Life Summit, Z Magazine 16, no. 4 (April), www.zmag.org.
13. UN Economic and Social Development Section, Population Division (2005), www.un.org; Economic Research Service, USDA (2005), www.ers.usda.gov.
14. W. C. Kim and R. Mauborgne (2005), *Blue Ocean Strategy: How to Create Uncontested Market Space and Make the Competition Irrelevant* (Boston: Harvard Business School Press).

Chapter 2
Globalization
What Caused It, and How Will It End?

Stephen J. Kobrin

What Is Globalization?

Globalization has been defined as "a hideous word of obscure meaning, coined in the 1960s, that came into ever-greater vogue in the 1990s."[1] While globalization may be a hideous word, it is in common use to imply both increased cross-border flows and economic, political, social, and cultural interconnectivity and integration. The first wave of globalization—characterized by dramatic increases in trade, investment, and migration—arose during the last third of the nineteenth century, faltered with the outbreak of World War I in 1914, and finally crashed on the shoals of the Great Depression in the early 1930s. The economic walls erected around national markets lasted for more than two decades, until the world economy began to reopen in the 1960s. The second or current wave of globalization emerged in the late 1980s with the end of the Cold War and the economic boom of the 1990s. Flows of trade and investment, and particularly the operations of multinational firms (foreign direct investment), expanded dramatically, and by the end of that decade globalization, especially in terms of an open world economy, was seen as the norm.

This brief excursion into economic history raises a question: will the second wave of globalization follow the path of the first? Is an open world economy epiphenomenal; is the open window about to slam shut once again? The signs in mid-decade are not encouraging. The Doha round of trade negotiations under the auspices of the World Trade Organization is in a coma and resuscitation looks problematic; there is increasing concern about investment by foreign multinationals in the United States and recent attempts to protect domestic firms as "national champions" in the EU; economic nationalism appears on the rise in Latin America; travel has gotten more difficult in the wake of the attacks on the World Trade Center; and, more generally, support for protectionism appears to be on the rise. It is reasonable to ask whether the dot-com crash of 2000 and the terrorist attacks of September 11, 2001, marked the end of an unusual period of economic openness, whether the second global economy is about to follow the path of the first.

Ending a story, however, requires development of a plot. Any discussion of the future trajectory of the second wave of globalization depends on how one accounts for its rise. One might suggest three different narratives with three different endings. First, globalization can be seen as cyclical: a function of the confluence of unusual economic and political conditions during the 1990s. Second, globalization could be a function of political will and political power. Last, it could be structural: a function of underlying technological change. While all three explanations are obviously interrelated, it is analytically useful to consider each in turn.

The Forms of Globalization

The 1990s were an unusual decade marked by the end of the Cold War and an economic boom driven by technology and the dot-com revolution. With the collapse of the Soviet Union, geopolitical and security issues receded and economics and wealth generation gained prominence, for states as well as for individuals and corporations. The dot-com boom and the opening of new markets in Eastern and Central Europe resulted in marked increases in levels of economic activity which in turn resulted in sharp increases in cross-border flows of trade and investment. The combination of the economic boom and reduced concerns about national security made it relatively easy for governments to lower—or even remove—barriers to flows of trade and investment. The result was an open global economy characterized by dramatic increases in flows of trade and investment, and particularly the international operations of multinational firms.

Globalization is a political act: opening borders to economic flows requires a positive act of will by government officials. From this perspective, the second wave of globalization can be explained as both the internationalization of the Reagan-Thatcher revolution and a reflection of the beliefs and interests of the United States as the dominant economic power. Globalization during the 1990s was a manifestation of the loss in faith in centrally managed economies after the collapse of the Soviet Union and the triumph of neoliberalism—the triad of deregulation, privatization, and openness to the international economy that came into vogue in both the United States and the UK during the 1980s. The United States, the dominant economic power during the decade, strongly believed in economic openness and put pressure on others to adopt it, both directly and indirectly through international organizations such as the World Bank. As the dominant power and the technological leader in an age of technology, the United States stood to benefit from free flows of trade and investment. The cliché that Great Britain's interests were reflected in the "imperialism of free trade" during the nineteenth century certainly applies to the United States one hundred years later. An open economy was in its interests: given America's superior competitive position, globalization's benefits greatly outweighed its costs.

The second wave of globalization can be seen as resulting from a technological revolution in transport and, especially, communication. In this case, jet transport and information technology dramatically changed the nature and the spatial scope of production. The Internet, email, and mobile phones allowed firms to link global operations in real time. The result was the internationalization of production and the disaggregation of supply chains. Firms began to break the entire process of product development, production, and distribution into bits and to distribute these "tasks" globally on the basis of efficiency. It has become increasing difficult to determine where a product was developed and produced. It is important to note that technology both facilitates globalization and increases the cost of economic autonomy or independence. The latter may be even more important than the former. Firms in strategic sectors such as pharmaceuticals, aerospace, semiconductors, and telecommunications are dependent on global markets to maintain a competitive research and development effort. In the 1930s, the cost of closing borders was a matter of degree. Most products could be replicated domestically, if at a higher cost. Given the globalization of research and development and reliance on disaggregated supply chains tied together through information technology, that is no longer true: the cost of replicating production of many products domestically would be prohibitive.

Conclusion

Each story has a different ending, perhaps many different endings. If you believe that globalization is cyclical, it is easy to point to the crash of 2000, the terrorist attacks of 9/11 (and the resulting "war on terror"), the sharp increase in oil prices and the scarcity of resources in general, and the resulting increase in protectionist politics and argue that the 1990s are over. The early years of the twenty-first century saw a marked downturn in the rate of growth of international trade and an absolute and very significant decline in the value of flows of foreign direct investment, which one would expect with a reduction in the level of economic activity. In some sense, economic and political conditions have returned to normal, with voters and their representatives concerned about job security and geopolitics once again rearing its ugly head. This narrative ends with the early twenty-first century marking the inflection point in the cycle and the start of a gradual—or perhaps not so gradual—closing of the world economy. A belief that globalization is political has some similar implications. The end of the boom of the 1990s affected the political will necessary to maintain open borders, with increased pressures on government officials to raise trade barriers (such as the U.S. steel tariffs of 2002), constrain inflows of foreign direct investment and protect national firms, restrict outsourcing of white collar jobs, and limit immigration. As important, the competitive position of the dominant power, the United States, changed dramatically. The rise of China and India as economic powers and the increasing technological sophistication of both countries have led to a reconsideration of the linkage between open borders and American interests. From a U.S. perspective, the benefit-cost ratio of economic openness has changed.

The third narrative, globalization as a function of underlying technological change, has a cloudier and less determinate ending. While changed economic and political conditions increase pressures on policy makers for protectionism, the cost of doing so over the medium to longer run may be prohibitive. Although technology does not determine economic and social relationships, it certainly limits the range of acceptable outcomes. The cost of trying to unwind the networks of multinational firms, reintegrating disaggregated supply chains, restricting the spatial scope of research and development efforts, or breaking up the Internet is simply too high to be tolerable. If you believe that the second wave of globalization is structural, there is no going back.

In reality, all three explanations are interrelated. However, globalization as a result of technological change dominates: in the medium to longer run, retreating to closed, autonomous national markets is not feasible economically. That is not necessarily good news: cyclical, political, and technological factors will all play a role in determining the future course of events. We are likely to face a dysfunctional global economy that we can neither escape nor make work for some time to come. Even though the costs of devolution may be too high to tolerate, pressures to protect domestic markets and resist international competition are not going to disappear. Dealing with these opposing forces will require multilateral cooperation and some form of effective and fair global economic governance.

At this point, as the collapse of the Doha round of trade negotiations indicates, effective and fair cooperative governance is in short supply. Globalization represents deep-seated and systemic change in the organization of economics and politics. The development of an effective multilateral system of governance will not be an easy or rapid process. Until that happens—and it could easily take decades—the interplay of cyclical, political, and technological forces is likely to result in a prolonged period of anxiety, uncertainty, and risk for everyone involved in the international economy.

Reference

1. M. Wolf (2004), *Why Globalization Works* (New Haven, Conn.: Yale University Press), 13.

Chapter 3
The Livestock Revolution and the Developing World

Cornelis de Haan and
Henning P. Steinfeld

The Demand for Livestock Products in Developing Countries

In recent years, across the world, there has been a 10 percent increase in land used for pastures, a 30 percent increase in cropland, a 79 percent increase in milk production (especially in South Asia), and a 230 percent increase in meat production (primarily poultry, pigs, and dairy, with poultry having the largest growth). Clearly, it is the livestock sector that has expanded the most, with East Asia taking the lead and Latin America second. A person in a developing country currently consumes half the amount of meat eaten by someone living in an industrialized country, but the global demand for livestock products is expected to double by 2050, with both demand for and the production of livestock products increasing faster in developing countries than in developed countries. Latin America is the major consumer of meat among developing countries but East Asia is catching up. Similarly, milk consumption in South Asia has increased substantially. Only Latin American countries are projected to have a sizable surplus of meat. All other developing countries will have a sizable deficit and will need to import. This is also true for milk and grain.

The factors that are driving increased demand in developing countries include changing demographics, urbanization, and income growth. Even in developing countries, the elderly population is increasing, and in general, older people eat more meat, milk and eggs. In addition, the human population will double by 2050 (we are adding around 75 million people every year to the global population). Eighty percent of the total growth is occurring in cities (much of it in the developing world), and people who live in cities tend to eat more meat. But higher incomes in developing countries are probably the most important factor driving the demand for meat and other livestock products. There is an emerging middle class in many populated, developing countries: people have become more affluent and more discerning in what they eat. This is particularly evident in East and South Asia, where population growth is the highest. However, some caveats are in order. For example, strong food taboos affect pork consumption in the Near East and North Africa and in Muslim countries. Beef is a food taboo in South Asia, Pakistan, and India, and large segments of the population in East Asia cannot digest milk and milk products because of lactose intolerance.

The Livestock Revolution and Structural Changes in the Livestock Sector

The large increase in demand for livestock products in the developing world and the emergence of production systems to meet that demand have been referred to as the "livestock revolution."[1] This revolution is based on expanding concentrate use, facilitated by the availability of cheap grains (more than one-third of the total grain production worldwide goes to feed animals), although oil cakes and roots and tubers are also important. By the year 2050, two billion tons of concentrates will be produced, compared to the 1.1 billion produced currently. The livestock revolution has also brought about major structural changes in the livestock sector in Asia and Latin America in terms of species composition, spatial distribution of production, and farm size. With respect to species composition, production in the monogastric pigs and poultry sector has grown much faster than production in the ruminant cattle and sheep sector. Although total meat production in developing countries more than tripled between 1980 and 2004, the growth in ruminant production was only 111 percent, while that of monogastrics expanded more than fourfold over the period.[2] With respect to spatial distribution, the location of pig and poultry production has become a more peri-urban activity, as demand in the towns grew faster than in the rural areas and transport economics (proximity to markets places and port) drove production closer to urban areas. Often, new production units are being built in areas where regulations are weak or not enforced. For example, pig and poultry production is highly concentrated around Bangkok in Thailand and around Hanoi and Ho Chi Minh City in Vietnam.[3] With respect to farm size, there has been large increase in the average size of the production unit in the pig and poultry sectors in many developing countries. For example, the percentage of poultry farms with more than 10,000 birds in Brazil increased from 52 percent to 73 percent over the period 1985–1999, and the percentage of pork from enterprises with more than five hundred animals in China increased from 8 percent to 40 percent over that same period.[4] Although many small producers are being squeezed out, the small-scale and backyard sector remains important. For example, in Indonesia in 2005, 39 percent of the poultry production still came from small commercial or backyard farms.[5] The continued importance of the small-scale and backyard sector also means that the marketing chain has maintained many traditional features, with a major share of the sales still occurring as live animals, in so-called wet markets, and most of the processing being carried out in small slaughterhouses.

At low levels of consumption, livestock products are a much desired and very important source of protein and micronutrients, particularly in areas where people suffer from malnutrition, and some of the structural changes that have arisen from the livestock revolution in developing countries are clearly beneficial. They have resulted in improvements in food safety and security: for example, vertical integration establishes closed food chains with quality control throughout. Similarly, supermarkets in the developing world are establishing their own quality standards. This process is driven by consumer demand for heightened standards for food quality, environmental stewardship, and animal welfare and is an example of a more general phenomenon in which private standards are beginning to take precedence over public standards.

On the other hand, increased livestock production threatens the environment. There is pollution due to gaseous by-products. For example, methane released from livestock systems (and from rice cultivation) and nitrous oxide released during the use of nitrogenous fertilizers together make up about 9 percent of the enhanced radiative forcing. Deforestation, as land is cleared for crops or pasture (especially in Latin America), biomass burning (including fuel wood), and other changes in land use practices release carbon dioxide, ammonia, and nitrous oxide into the atmosphere; these activities together account for about 18 percent of the enhanced radiative forcing. There is increased water use. Domestic animals drink only about 1 percent of all the water used, but crop irrigation, especially crops grown to feed animals, account for about 15 percent of all the water used, and because many of the water catchment areas in the world are pasture areas upstream, livestock also have an important impact on water harvesting, as well as on the water cycle in general. Finally, soil erosion and pesticide use and encroachments on wildlife habitat continue to increase. We can gauge how this might affect the developing world by considering the situation in the United States, where 55 percent of the erosion, 37 percent of the pesticides, and 32 percent of the nitrogen and phosphorus originate from the livestock sector in one way or another, that is, from livestock production itself or from feed production. The search for greater efficiency in the competition for feed resources, which was the main driver for the fast growth in the pig and poultry sectors, has also encouraged the use of growth promoters and other feed additives, creating a major risk to public health through antibiotic resistance and the discharge of heavy metals into the environment. In addition, contact between animals and humans has increased dramatically. Around most major cities in Asia and Latin America (and to a limited extent in Africa), there is now a very high concentration of monogastric livestock farms; the animals are kept under a variety of farming systems, and they are sold mostly in open markets and processed in slaughterhouses and through retail systems with poor sanitary control systems. As the number of production units in peri-urban surroundings increases, so also will opportunities for the emergence of new infectious diseases, especially in areas where regulation is weak or unenforced. The close proximity of animal housing to people provides ideal conditions for the emergence of disease (Nipah virus, SARS, and highly pathogenic avian influenza). Over the past decade, the threat of emerging and reemerging diseases has increased. It is exacerbated by the growing international trade in animal products and the increased international movement of people, both of which facilitate the rapid dissemination of pathogens and complicate their containment. Finally, the increased consumption of livestock products may lead to increases in the incidence of obesity and cardiovascular disease in the developing world.

Institutional Framework and Veterinary Services

These risks to global public health have occurred against a background of weakened public veterinary control systems in most developing countries, which were unprepared to face the exponential growth of the pig and poultry system. These services traditionally have focused on single diseases of ruminant systems, without taking a broader view. In addition, these services, especially in transition economies and in Latin America, experienced significant budget cuts at the same time they were charged with more responsibilities in areas such as diseases of production (metabolic diseases, mastitis), food safety and international trade, and the fast-growing aquaculture sector. The situation is exacerbated by complex, shifting, and sometimes ad hoc service arrangements. Considerable efforts over the past decades by international agencies and some national governments to arrive at a better distribution of responsibilities between public and private veterinarians and between professional and paraprofessional agents have not produced the hoped-for result. In many developing countries in sub-Saharan Africa and South Asia, vested interests have caused public sector veterinarians to continue to provide private clinical services to individual animals. As a result, the public services are stretched too thin in providing public good services, such as control of major epizootic diseases, food safety control, and other control functions. The continued involvement by public veterinary agents in clinical work also stifles the emergence of a private veterinary profession, which could carry out these functions more efficiently. At the same time, however, professional veterinarians are reluctant to delegate responsibilities to paraprofessionals, who could provide a more affordable and more efficient service to smallholders and pastoralists.[6] Public veterinarians apparently fear the competition more than they appreciate the synergies between these two professional levels, as demonstrated in several countries.

Simultaneously, many developing countries have gone through a period of decentralization of responsibilities from national to provincial (state) and district level. While decentralization was initiated to increase the voice of the people at the grassroots level, it is not clear whether transferring authority to a regional or community level was advisable in the case of animal health, for national interests often must take precedence over local ones in matters of quarantine, early alerts, and early responses. Moreover, veterinary services in many countries, especially in sub-Saharan Africa, were integrated into general agricultural research and extension services, thereby avoiding creation of the special structures necessary to control animal diseases and safeguard public health. As a result of all these forces, the authority of the veterinary services has declined significantly, and that in turn has affected their independence in disease reporting. As became evident in the recent outbreaks of SARS and highly pathogenic influenza, reporting is often delayed because of political and economic vested interests. In short, public animal health services, often underfunded and weakened in their authority, operating under cumbersome lines of command, and maintaining inappropriate work priorities, are facing major changes in the structure of the livestock industry that are causing new, poorly known risks to animal and human health.

The Way Forward

There is a need for urgent action at all levels. At the international level, there is a need to recognize animal health as a global public good, acknowledging the spillover of diseases from a particular country to a whole region, or even the world. For this reason, it is in the direct interest of the developed world to support improved disease control in the developing world. For example, the foot-and-mouth disease outbreak of 2001, which caused the UK economy an estimated U.S. $8 billion loss, originated in Southeast Asia. An investment of industrial nations in animal disease surveillance and early alert systems in Southeast Asia might have contained the disease and prevented this tremendous loss to the UK economy. A new look at how animal disease surveillance is organized, reported, and financed is therefore needed.

Although there are clearly international public goods involved in the control of animal disease, developing countries are not absolved of their responsibilities. Here we must consider that developing countries are not all at the same point in economic structural change; the stage of development of each country's economy in general and its livestock sector in particular will define to a major extent what needs to be done to make the sector more sustainable and safer. Countries with a well-developed export sector, such as Thailand, or with a growing middle class, such as India, need different animal health and food safety policies than countries with mostly poor rural consumers. Nevertheless, we can make some key general policy recommendations. First, it is important to restore the balance between animal waste production and the absorptive capacity of the surrounding land.[4] This will have beneficial effects on the environment, reduce disease transmission risks, and possibly open up opportunities for smallholders, who are now in the danger of being crowded out by the industrial sector. Possible mechanisms to this end include adjusting the spatial distribution of livestock operations (through tax incentives based on the distance from urban areas). It is also important to try to improve the efficiency of feed and energy use (in Europe, major reductions can be made in nitrate and phosphate loading in surface water and groundwater through improvements in feed conversion and appropriate incentives for reducing biogas). Second, veterinary services—in particular, early detection, alert, and response systems—should be strengthened to ensure the independence of disease reporting, support the preparation of disease preparedness plans (which includes providing compensation funds), and improve diagnostic capability through regional networks. Third, the relevance of formal food safety standards should be assessed and priority diseases defined on the basis of human health hazards, trade prospects, and cost-benefit analyses. Food safety standards should also consider the appropriate requirements for domestic markets, where food preparation habits are often different, and the Codex-based, so-called gold standards of the industrial world. The imposition of international gold standards on products intended for local consumption could well make the products out of reach for the poor, and the use of a parallel set of standards, one for export markets and one for local markets, might be preferable. The milk market in Nairobi provides an example: raw milk is sold locally but is boiled before consumption by 96 percent of households. After boiling, this milk has a lower pathogen count than pasteurized milk obtained in the formal sector.

Fourth, a better distribution of responsibilities is necessary between public and private services and between professional and paraprofessional veterinary agents so that the vested interests, which till now have affected the efficiency of the national and international services, are eliminated. This includes the public service sector restricting its activities to providing the public services of surveillance and control of zoonoses and diseases of trade, food safety, and quality control, with the private veterinary sector focusing on clinical services and executing subcontracts of public services. A similar division of labor can also be envisaged between professional and paraprofessional veterinarians in areas where professional clinical practices are financially no longer attractive.

Conclusion

The livestock revolution will continue, driven by an increase in the global demand for meat.[7] In the developing world in particular the demand for meat and milk will continue to grow. This increasing demand for livestock products will bring about new challenges for the veterinary profession. A major challenge is mitigating the negative environmental and public health effects of vastly increased livestock numbers in closer contiguity to humans. Other challenges include reducing vested interests in the delivery of veterinary services, arriving at a better definition of global, national, and private responsibilities, and increasing funding to address the global challenges. There are major policy and institutional gaps to be remediated before the desired objectives can be achieved. Veterinary education is a major tool in this battle. For veterinary schools in the developed world, this might mean more attention to the development of curricula addressing these issues in a holistic fashion and an expanded teaching program to include course work aimed at paraprofessionals and veterinary economists. Veterinary education must focus on promoting interdisciplinary work that looks at production systems and the food chain from an economic and ecosystem prospective.

In addition to a shift in scientific perspective, veterinarians need to strengthen their information management skills and develop methods for working on interdisciplinary team. "Soft" skills such as awareness building and public relations management should be included in the curriculum. With a more ecosystem-oriented scientific base and better knowledge of communications, veterinarians will be in excellent position to understand and affect global issues related to controlling epidemics, herd health, and food safety and quality. The new consumers of the coming decades will want pathogen-free, residue-free meat and milk, and resistance to bioengineered products may spread. As a result, veterinary practitioners, scientists, and economists should be capable of addressing global issues associated with increased production in the developing world.

References

1. C. Delgado, M. Rosengrant, H. Steinfeld, S. Ehui, and C. Courbois (1999), "Livestock to 2020: The Next Food Revolution," Discussion Paper 28 (Washington, D.C.: International Food Policy Research Center).

2. H. Steinfeld, P. Gerber, T. Wassenaar, V. Castel, M. Rosales, and C. de Haan (2006), *Livestock's Long Shadow: Environmental Issues and Options* (Rome: FAO).

3. P. Gerber, P. Chilonda, G. Franceschini, and H. Menzi (2005), "Geographical Determinants and Environmental Implications of Livestock Production Intensification in Asia," *Bioresource Technology* 96: 263–76.

4. World Bank (2005), *Managing the Livestock Revolution* (Washington, D.C.: World Bank).

5. World Bank (2006), Enhancing Control of Highly Pathogenic Avian Influenza in Developing Countries Through Compensation, World Bank Technical Paper, Agriculture and Rural Development Department (Washington, D.C.: World Bank).

6. A. Catley, T. Leyland, J. C. Mariner, D. M. O. Akabwai, B. Admassu, W. Asfaw, G. Bekele, B. Admassu, and H. S. Hassan (2004), "Para-Veterinary Professionals and the Development of Quality, Self Sustaining Community Based Services," *OIE Review of Science and Technology* 23, no. 1: 225–52.

7. *New York Times* (2006), Editorial, December 27.

Chapter 4
Technology, Innovation, Research, and Development

David T. Galligan and Edward Kanara

Modern animal agriculture production systems are the consequence of human evolution in the discovery and implementation of technologies throughout the ages. Local resources are used in combination with appropriate technologies to produce products that are desired by society yet sufficiently priced to ensure economic and environmental sustainability of the operation. Which technologies are implemented in a given geographic region depends on a number of factors, including the availability and cost of input resources, competing opportunities for alternative use of these inputs, the proximity of markets for the products produced, societal affluence, and local cultural and social attitudes toward animal agriculture. New technologies will continue to change how humans interact with food animals and ultimately will define the structure of our animal production industries. In this chapter we discuss fundamental structural changes occurring in animal production systems and the economic basis for these changes.

General History of Technological Evolution in Animal Agriculture

Technology in its broadest definition is an improvement in the allocation of limited resources for a stated purpose. The cost and risk associated with the implementation of the technology must be off-set in value by the improved production. Efficient animal production of foodstuffs ensures a nation's supply of stable, safe, highly valued nutrients. It is a vital component of the food security portfolio of a nation and, when highly efficient, allows society to pursue other activities of value.[1,2]

The very act of animal domestication, estimated to have occurred approximately 13,000 years ago, is one of the most important technological advances of mankind. Through this step and the adoption of various associated technologies over time, the resulting improved availability and predictability of food brought great benefits to societies. Animal domestication was a catalyst for other advances and helps to explain the historical emergence of cultures in various regions of the world.[1] In these early stages, advances can be measured in the domestication of additional species. Of the world's 148 terrestrial mammalian herbivores and omnivores weighing more than 45 kg, only fourteen have been domesticated.[1] It is doubtful that additional species will be domesticated for food consumption in the future. Later advances took the form of managing animals in larger herds and controlling major devastating diseases. In fact, the formation of the first veterinary school, in Lyons, France, in 1762, occurred in response to the massive losses of cattle to rinderpest. Early concepts in animal segregation, along with basic principles of sanitation such as the Lancisi edicts of 1714, were used to help control outbreaks and became the foundation of modern biosecurity practices. Continued advances in veterinary medicine, housing, ventilation, vaccines, milking machines, culling management, RFID technology, feed management systems, and herd management systems have allowed even greater aggregation of animals. Over time, improvements in yield per animal unit have also been realized through better animal nutrition and management. While some of this increase in yield has occurred through improved genetics and the selection of animals with specific valued traits, it is also due to the implementation of technologies. For example, the dairy industry in the United States has seen a reduction in total cow numbers (22 million in 1950 to 9 million in 2006), increased total milk yield, increased yield per cow (a 3.6-fold increase from 1950), decreased farm numbers, and increased number of cows per farm. Many of the technologies that have allowed animal aggregation—nutrition management, better housing, disease control—have also enhanced production yields.

The fundamental economic basis of these trends toward larger herd size and increased yield per animal unit is the realization of higher returns when fixed costs, such as labor per capital, are spread over more units of product and variable costs are pursued as long as the marginal revenue is greater then the marginal cost. These concepts are best visualized as a simple graph whose shape defines the state of technology in converting inputs to outputs. Fixed costs are those costs that will not change over the immediate planning horizon and thus are horizontal. Variable costs are directly associated with production and, when added to fixed costs, yield the total cost of production for a given level of input. Greatest returns occur when the product value minus total cost is maximal. It is the point at which the marginal cost (variable) and marginal revenue are equal, giving rise to the principle of marginal returns. This simple principle is behind many of the structural changes that have occurred in animal agriculture over time. Herds and flocks have increased in size, such that fixed costs are spread over more animal units and ultimately over more products. Yield per animal unit has increased to spread animal maintenance costs (and replacement costs) over more units of production. The curves change in magnitude as society changes the values of inputs and outputs, and the shape of the curve changes when technologies are regulated or changed. All technologies were at one point in time variable inputs to animal production, and those with favorable economic margins were embraced and became fixed over time, defining standard production practices for a region. In fact, a successful technology can be defined as an input that was once variable to an industry and is now a fixed cost.

We can illustrate how this works using the example of bovine somatotropin (BST). This example serves not only to illustrate the economic principles outlined earlier but also to introduce a broader discussion of the role of the animal health industry in developing and introducing new technologies. BST is a relatively recent recombinant DNA technology product whose history of development is surrounded by controversy in terms of the production impacts on the dairy industry, as well as its safety to animals and humans. The Food and Drug Administration (FDA) and U.S. Department of Agriculture (USDA) approved the use of BST in 1993 after an extensive evaluation period and a contentious review process; however, the controversy is not over. It is an interesting technology in that the production responses are quick, significant (approximately 10 lb/cow/day), measurable, and scale neutral in terms of implementation. These marginal pounds of milk per cow are highly profitable (100–300 percent return per invested implementation cost) in that the only investment by the producer is in the product ($.47/day) and the additional feed the cow consumes in making the milk (approximately $.03 of additional feed/lb milk response). The animals' maintenance costs are fixed and independent of production. This additional milk capacity can be viewed as: "sitting on the shelf": it is not at risk of contracting disease, does not require additional cows to produce or their replacements, does not require additional barn capacity and the resulting manure holding capacity, and so on. It is estimated that if BST were to be removed from use by the dairy industry in the United States, approximately 313,372 more adult lactating cows and 246,015 replacement heifers —equivalent to more than half the dairy industry of Pennsylvania— would have to be added to the current national herd of 9 million. These additional animals would conservatively require a land mass of 610,931 acres (1.4 acres/cow and 0.7 acres/heifer, for phosphorus balance), which is approximately 37 percent of the acreage of Yellowstone National Park or 87 percent of the acreage of Yosemite National Park.

Research and Development in the Animal Health Industry and the Adoption of New Technologies

The animal health industry, here considered to comprise the manufacturers of veterinary medicines, vaccines, and other animal health products, is an important agent of innovation. In 2005, global animal health sales were about $15 billion, and the top fifteen companies accounted for about 80 percent of those sales. Growth in sales has been rather flat over the past several years. Even so, between 2002 and 2005 the animal health industry increased its spending on research and development by 8 to 10 percent. There are several opportunities for the animal health industry. It is well-known that food-borne illnesses have a tremendous impact on public health, and there is some interesting innovative work going on right now in terms of vaccines for cattle, swine, and poultry that are intended to decrease bacterial shedding in animals infected by pathogens that may threaten human health (*Salmonella, Campylobacter,* and *Escherichia coli* O157). The economic challenge presented by such vaccines is the question of who will pay for them. Producers have to believe it is worth investing in a vaccine that may not materially improve the productivity of their stock, that they will realize more profit from their livestock by vaccinating than by not vaccinating. Currently there is very little incentive to adopt a technology like this. Perhaps this will change as private standards take precedence over public standards (see Chapter 3) and consumers (and the slaughter and packing industry) demand that livestock farmers do something to decrease the risk of food-borne disease.

Even animal diseases that do not directly affect humans present difficult therapeutic challenges. For example, the USDA estimates that in 2006, the cattle industry will lose $2 billion due to bovine respiratory disease (BRD). While it is incumbent on the animal health industry to make sure we are continuously replacing and working on the next generation of anti-infectives for diseases like BRD, there is an overarching mandate that we also encourage the responsible, prudent, and judicious use of the antimicrobial products that emerge. The challenge is fairly straightforward: we need to be able to treat food animal disease without jeopardizing the ability of antimicrobials to treat disease in people. With respect to antimicrobials, the goal is responsible development, responsible use, and responsible monitoring. Human health must be the first priority of the animal health industry. The FDA states that antimicrobials are considered safe if there is reasonable certainty of no harm to human health from the proposed use of the drug in food animals. In 2003, the FDA introduced Guidance 152, which describes a process in which a proposed antimicrobial product undergoes a risk assessment based on three components: a release assessment, which determines the probability that resistant bacteria will be present in animals as a result of antimicrobial use; an exposure assessment, which gauges the likelihood that humans will ingest resistant bacteria; and a consequences assessment, which assesses the chances that human exposure to the resistant bacteria would result in adverse human health consequences. Based on that information, an overall risk estimation of high, medium, or low is arrived at, and the FDA uses this information in its determination of whether that drug is to be approved or not and, if it is approved, under what conditions it may be used. The animal health industry itself also has a direct impact on whether or not drugs are used responsibly. For example, recent antimicrobial advertisements in magazines and journals intended for farmers included no discussion of the attributes of the drug being advertised (the only reference to the drug was the label, which was printed in the body of the advertisement). Instead, the focus of the narrative was about responsible use. Points of emphasis included the importance of the relationship between the client and the veterinarian, appropriate dosing, appropriate duration of dosing, and the importance of using drugs in food animals precisely as the label directs. There was also a commentary about the consequences of failure to adhere to the principles of responsible use.

Forces That Promote Collaborative Efforts for the Development of New Technologies

The emergence or reemergence of infectious diseases such as West Nile virus, leptospirosis, and Lyme disease has long been a major factor in promoting collaborative efforts between the animal health industry and other stakeholders. However, highly pathogenic avian influenza has been almost unique in its ability to energize and bring together the relevant groups. For example, the International

Federation for Animal Health, an organization representing manufacturers of veterinary medicines, vaccines, and other animal health products in both developed and developing countries across five continents, has consulted with the World Health Organization, the Food and Agriculture Organization, the OIE, and the EU to develop a consensus for action. In the United States, the animal health industry works through the Animal Health Institute, which consults on a regular basis with both the USDA and the Centers for Disease Control. A consensus has evolved that the industry should focus on protecting poultry health to reduce the likelihood of an avian influenza epidemic in poultry and to preserve the availability of chicken eggs for the production of human influenza vaccines. Another potential motivation for collaboration is the threat of agroterrorism. Possible industry roles here include medical prophylaxis, advanced medical countermeasures, and improved diagnostic capabilities. Nevertheless, the animal health industry faces some considerable obstacles in this regard. As Noreen Hynes, Director of Research and Development Coordination for the Department of Human Services, so succinctly put it, "The incentive is not there for large pharmaceutical companies." The problems include the uncertainty of developing a product that may never be used, uncertainty about what might be an appropriate charge for a product meeting a genuine national security need, and product liability issues.

Conclusion

The history of agriculture is a story of the implementation of technologies. This history has allowed societies to pursue other interests that advance the greater good of a community. To be embraced by the animal industry, the technology must offer the producer an appropriate return relative to the costs and associated risks, as well as being acceptable to consumers. Although the nature of the technology has changed over time, it has spawned two general phenomena in the animal production industries: increased consolidation and dramatic improvements in production yields per animal. Both of these trends dilute fixed costs by spreading them over more units of production. To meet the demand for animal products associated with population growth and the upward shift in consumption of animal food products in developing world populations, existing technologies will need to be more broadly adopted and new technologies developed. The modern animal health industry has been a major force for innovation and the adoption of new technology, and is increasingly working in collaboration with other stakeholders. Nevertheless, even when there is a clear and major public good to be achieved, it is not always obvious what incentives might encourage the industry to become involved. Society in general must balance, on many dimensions, the trade-offs associated with the adoption or nonadoption of technologies.

References

1. J. Diamond (2002),"Evolution, Consequences and Future of Plant and Animal Domestication," *Nature* 418: 700–707.

2. D. Avery (2000), *Saving the Planet with Pesticides and Plastic*, 2nd ed. (Indianapolis: Hudson Institute).

Chapter 5
Animal Welfare in Livestock Production
Implications for Producers,
Consumers, and Public Health

Paul B. Thompson

After decades of resistance to the urgings of animal protection-
ists, livestock producers are currently undertaking a variety of initiatives to improve the welfare of animals in their care. Some of
the changes are best described as evolutionary, including revi-
sions to longstanding husbandry guidelines promulgated by producer, veterinary, and animal science organizations, while others
represent wholly new ventures in the form of collaborations with
animal advocates to formulate husbandry standards for products
marketed to consumers on the basis of superior husbandry. The
process of change should itself be viewed against a backdrop of
longstanding beliefs among veterinarians about the nature of animal welfare and their ethical responsibilities to the animals under
their care. This chapter briefly examines what is happening and
why, then identifies some of the challenges on the horizon. The
primary focus is on farm production methods and the husbandry
associated with those practices, and the discussion is limited to
the United States and Canada. I argue that changes in the supply
chain for food animal production in North America over the past

two centuries have brought us to the current situation and set the stage for future challenges.

Livestock Husbandry Around 1800

The term *livestock* implies the human use of domesticated animals as sources of food, fiber, and in some settings mechanical energy for the performance of household tasks. Excluded are domesticated animals such as cats and dogs, even when these animals are maintained in human households because of their utility in performing tasks such as household security, hunting, herding, or controlling vermin. We are thus reminded that the categories we use to characterize animals and our relationships to them are shot through with somewhat arbitrary meanings that have accrued over generations of practice and discourse. Ambiguity surrounding the expression "animal welfare" is of more recent and of rational origin, as there have been numerous attempts over the past century to specify those aspects of animals and their lives that are the primary focus of our obligations to them. With respect to livestock, *husbandry* is particularly relevant to any specification of welfare, as it is the traditional word for characterizing appropriate forms and practices of animal care.

One useful way to summarize much of the change that has occurred in livestock production is to focus on the supply chain that extends between primary animal producers—farmers and ranchers—and consumers of animal products. There was a time in North American history when this chain was very short indeed— perhaps forty or fifty feet from the barnyard to the kitchen. We may pick the year 1800 as an arbitrary anchor point for our history of animal production. At this point, approximately 80 percent of European settlers would have been primarily engaged in farming, and their farm operations, together with hunting and scavenging, would have supplied most of their needs for animal products, especially food needs. Many Americans would have been engaged in a number of additional enterprises besides farming, and those who did not farm at all would very likely have obtained most of their animal products from neighbors who were known to them personally. A few more extended supply chains existed, especially in the burgeoning textile sector, where supply chains for cotton, silk, and flax were already operating on a global scale. But for animal products, and especially food products, the source animals would typically have been raised in the same locales in which they were consumed in the form of milk, meat, eggs, hides, and other by-products.

Can we characterize the thinking of producers and consumers regarding the ethics of husbandry for the period around 1800? The main philosophical positions were certainly in print by this time, with René Descartes (1596–1650) and Immanuel Kant (1724–1804) having argued that the key question is whether animals have the degree of rationality required for language. Both answered the question negatively. Descartes implies that animals are machines, in this way justifying our use of them, while Kant develops the more subtle view that our duties to animals are indirect, reflecting aspects of our own moral character rather than respect for them as moral subjects. On the opposite side were philosophers such as Voltaire (1694–1778) and Jeremy Bentham (1748–1832), the latter of whom offered the most succinct riposte in his 1789 work, *The Principles of Morals and Legislation*: "the question is not, Can they reason? nor, Can they talk? but, Can they suffer?"

We cannot presume that American farmers would have been aware of this philosophical debate, though Thomas Jefferson writes in one of his letters that it is very likely many would have read some philosophy. There are farm diaries and agrarian tracts from this period, but they make infrequent references to animals. We may discern from this that livestock husbandry was not regarded as particularly worthy of note. This may mean, on the one hand, that those who took the trouble to write on farm issues did not see husbandry as an important ethical practice. On the other hand, it may mean they did not regard the condition of animals as ethically problematic. What seems most likely is that the owners of livestock were thought to have an ethical responsibility to provide good husbandry, but that this responsibility was held to be entirely consistent with human self-interest. Animals that were faring poorly would not be serving the purposes for which they were being kept in the first place.

How would we today evaluate animal welfare in each of the three domains of animal bodies, minds, and natures? Animals in 1800 were raised primarily in extensive conditions, with occasional husbandry. Human husbandry consisted largely of herding animals to sources of food and water, and in some cases bringing feed to them. There would have been some attention to calving or lambing, but for the most part these animals were on their own. They were exposed to the elements and to predators, though owners of livestock would have attempted to limit death from predation. The animals received virtually no veterinary care and would have been vulnerable to health problems related to injury, exposure, and diseases acquired from wildlife and other livestock, though relatively low population densities would have shielded them from some mechanisms of animal disease transmission. As such, it seems reasonable to rank welfare on the scale of animal bodies as relatively low. On the other hand, livestock living under such conditions (with the possible exception of poultry) would have engaged in most natural behaviors in order to reproduce and survive. Hence we may rank welfare on the animal natures scale as relatively high. I confess I do not know what to say about animal minds in 1800. Certainly the health and environmental conditions must have introduced some level of stress and discomfort, so perhaps we should simply rate this in the middle range.

Livestock Husbandry Around 1900

If we fast-forward 100 years, we see significant changes in the supply chain for animal products, but much less significant change in on-farm husbandry or attitudes. By 1900, industrialization and urban growth had taken hold on the east coast of North America. This created a demand for meat, milk, and animal product supply chains that extended far into the interior, serviced first by shipping routes over water and later by railroads. This infrastructure in turn spawned the growth of Midwestern cities, which served as hubs for this supply chain. Animal slaughter and processing was critical to the growth of several cities during the years leading up to our arbitrary century mark, including Cincinnati (known as Porkopolis), Chicago, and Kansas City. Thus, there were now a number of actors inserted between primary producers and consumers of animal products, including those involved in transport, slaughter, processing, and retailing to urban consumers. Although generalizations are tricky, it is nonetheless accurate to say that the greatest concentration and dominance of large-scale enterprise in this supply chain occurred in the middle. Railroads and processors rapidly became very large firms that could exert substantial control over smaller and economically less well-organized animal producers, and retailers also tended to be small, independently owned markets, butchers, and restaurateurs.

One additional aspect of the supply chain bears mention. By 1900, many of the key elements for an agricultural supply industry were starting to take shape, especially in connection with the development of milling and feed supply. Railroads and grain elevators were critical to the emergence of a consolidated global grain industry. The primary markets for commodity grain were human consumption and provisioning animals during their relatively short stays in stockyards awaiting shipment and slaughter. However, unlike the supply chain in 1800, it was now possible to purchase animal feeds from centralized suppliers, and the input side of animal production would become increasingly important throughout the twentieth century. A structure of agricultural machinery inputs was also being built, though at this point equipment was primarily focused on crop production. The key point is that on-farm production of crops and animals was not the start of the supply chain even in 1900, as farmers and ranchers were becoming increasingly dependent on suppliers themselves.

Relative to 1800, the circumstances bearing on animals' lives were changed dramatically during transport and slaughter, those phases of the supply chain that were undergoing the processes of industrialization. Descriptions of the early stockyards and slaughterhouses depict conditions in which all three dimensions of animal welfare must have rated very low, though the relatively short duration of these conditions may have prevented animal health issues from manifesting to the extent they would have, had animals remained in transit or in stockyards for very long. Such conditions were terrible for both animals and humans, inducing Upton Sinclair to write *The Jungle* in 1906. This in turn led to the passage of the Pure Food and Drug Act and the creation of government regulations for health and safety in the United States. The first U.S. statute on animal cruelty dealt with transport and was passed in 1877.

On-farm, however, changes in animal husbandry were less dramatic. The changes in the animal industry during the nineteenth century suggest that by 1900, animal production was being thought of as a commercial enterprise on many farms and ranches, as opposed to a domestic activity intended to provision the family and a few neighbors. There were a number of animal producers who definitely thought of themselves as commercial producers, especially in the wool industry and the Western cattle industry. Yet a great deal of animal production still occurred on diversified farms, where several species of animals might be raised in parallel with predominantly crop production activities. Whether in specialized or diversified operations, most animals were kept under extensive conditions, with access to pasture or barnyard whenever weather conditions permitted. Veterinary medical assistance was beginning to become more widely available. Classes in veterinary medicine had been offered since the end of the Civil War. The College of Veterinary Medicine at Cornell University opened its doors in 1894. As such, it seems reasonable to conclude that prior to transport and slaughter, the quality of welfare for farm animals was not markedly different from 1800 to 1900, with the possibility that with improving veterinary care, there were attendant improvements on the dimension of animal bodies.

Awareness of problems associated with transport and slaughter indicates that for some Americans at least, animal welfare was coming to be seen as a potential problem. Furthermore, the use of draft animals outside the farm had expanded with the growth of industrial production, and the treatment of horses was often abysmal in these conditions. Animal protection initiatives were beginning to promote better treatment of horses and to protest the treatment of livestock during transport and while being held for slaughter. These facts indicate that in at least some quarters of American agriculture, animal interests were sacrificed for monetary profits. Farmers and ranchers cannot have been wholly ignorant of the conditions their animals would have to endure after crossing the farm gate on their way to Eastern dinner plates. Nevertheless, the on-farm ethic of husbandry would still have held that good care of animals was wholly consistent with the interests of the farmer. Furthermore, although the passage of a law to protect animals in transport acknowledges a role for state action on behalf of animals, animal husbandry was still regarded as a personal responsibility of the producer.

In conclusion, although it would be decidedly mistaken to see the agrarian past as a golden age for livestock ethics, it is nonetheless accurate to see it as a time when few considered on-farm husbandry as a key locus for ethical problems in the relationship between animals and human beings. Although some important developments for animal welfare were associated with industrialization in the nineteenth century, they did not have dramatic or even predominantly adverse impacts on the conditions under which livestock lived the largest part of their lives on farms and ranches. Husbandry was regarded as an ethical responsibility that keepers of livestock owed to the animals under their care, but it was also regarded as a responsibility that rested lightly on the shoulders of farmers and ranchers as a result of the perceived consonance between animal health and well-being, on the one hand, and producer economic incentives on the other. While the first inklings of animal care as a broader social concern are perceptible, husbandry ethics were not seen as the responsibility of consumers or other actors in the supply chain.

The Current Situation

By 2000, changes that were afoot in 1900 had developed in ways that dramatically altered the supply chain for meat, milk, eggs, and animal by-products. Overall, farming of all kinds has shifted to specialized production systems. Production systems that involve both crops and livestock still exist, but they are no longer the norm. In the main, farmers grow crops, which they sell to different farmers, who feed livestock. Furthermore, livestock operations are specialized: beef producers are not dairymen, dairy owners do not produce eggs or broilers, and none of them produce pigs. A supply chain that was once not obviously a chain at all is now a clear progression of distinct production processes coupled in series by economic transactions of one sort or another. Consumers, at an extreme end of this chain, generally have little knowledge of the source or supply organization of the animal products they consume.

It is certainly the case that the consolidation evident with the processing industry, well under way in 1900, has continued, creating systems of vertical integration in which companies such as Tyson Foods have extended their control in both directions. At the consumer end, such companies offer branded products to consumers through supermarkets. At the other end, companies contract with producers (who are increasingly referred to as "growers" or "feeders") to deliver animals ready for processing on strict schedules. In many cases, the people once known as farmers do not even own the animals, though they do typically own the production facilities and assume a great deal of the financial risk associated with livestock and poultry production during the interval when the animals are under their care. Often, the feed, husbandry, and veterinary care made available to animals are specified in these contracts to a level of detail that limits the decision making of producers considerably. There is, however, considerable variability in the organization of animal production on both a species and a regional basis, with poultry exhibiting the greatest amount of integration and beef cattle continuing to have a large number of independent owner-operators who sell animals to feedlots for finishing.

Two less well-known but crucial aspects of the supply chain must be noted. At the supply end, consolidation in the grain industry has conspired with many decades of subsidy payments to producers of commodity grains such as corn and soybeans. It is very inexpensive to deliver an entire trainload of animal feed to a single location and to sell it at rate that may be below the cost of production. The result is that feeding animals in large numbers in proximity to railheads is often cheaper than allowing animals to graze on rangeland or pasture, even though forage from range and pasture is often the product of rainfall, sunshine, and the natural fertility of soils and grasses. When coupled to consolidation in processing, this aspect of the contemporary supply chain has proved to be a powerful force encouraging the clustering of concentrated animal feeding operations, or CAFOs, within specific regions and a corresponding decline in competitiveness of extensive animal production, especially on diversified family-owned farms.

The clustering of CAFOs has been the source of great controversy in animal production. While these production systems score as well as and often better than traditional animal husbandry on standard veterinary health measures, confining animals indoors on concrete or in cages has been widely criticized by animal protection organizations. These criticisms often focus on crowding or housing conditions that limit animals' ability to engage in natural behavior and very likely cause mental frustration, distress, fear, and possibly boredom. As such, the current situation is one in which improvements in welfare in the domain of animal bodies are entirely offset by declines in welfare in the domains of animal minds and animal natures. Furthermore, when maintenance and basic husbandry suffer in these settings, sometimes through equipment failure or human error, situations referred to in the industry as a "train wreck" can have catastrophic consequences for the welfare of many animals at one time.

What is more, when many animals are confined together, disposal of animal waste becomes difficult. Individual CAFOs have developed systems for holding wastes in lagoons, but lagoon systems have been subject to flooding and leakage, which has created serious pollution issues in some cases. Even in the best of situations, CAFOs are associated with noxious odors, and when they are developed in clusters, air and water pollution can become ongoing problems. Furthermore, this system of production disrupts ecological nitrogen cycles, which brings into question the long-term ecological sustainability of this approach to animal production. On top of animal welfare, pollution, and sustainability, clusters have also been associated with social disruption in a number of settings, as both physical and social infrastructure in local communities may be inadequate to service industrial facilities manned by low-wage workers who are newcomers to the local community.

The second change in supply chains is on the consumer end, as very large integrated retailers have emerged during the last twenty-five years in both the grocery and restaurant sector. In both cases, between ten and fifteen companies control the majority of sales in animal products, and firms such as Wal-Mart or McDonald's Corporation may control significant fractions of retail sales in their sector alone. As such, these companies have significant market power to insist on standards from suppliers. What is more, the growth in standards has exploded over the last decade in particular, as new food safety–based standards have been applied both in the United States and globally and as standards requiring farm-to-grocery-shelf tracking of meats have been imposed in Europe. Other standards are voluntary and have been developed either for inventory control or to create high-value markets for products, such as USDA Certified Organic, or, in the animal products industry, meats, milk, and eggs labeled as nutritionally enhanced or produced under circumstances that promise higher levels of welfare.

These changes at the consumer end of the supply chain have also resulted in a number of efforts to develop industrywide standards in animal production, mostly focused on animal welfare. The best known of these efforts was initiated by McDonald's, which has used its supplier contracting to enforce standards calling for greater space for birds in egg-laying facilities and for pigs in pork production. This effort was quickly followed by Burger King, and industrywide standards have been pursued in recent years by a trade group, the National Chain Restaurant Association. As such, changes in supply chains have both created the impetus for clusters of CAFOs and at the same time have created extragovernmental means for enforcing standards on animal production methods.

Chapter 6
Animal Plagues
The Political and Economic Consequences of Nonzoonotic Animal Diseases

Gary Smith

Disease epidemics in domestic animals can have profound effects on the health and well-being of human populations. Only a minority of the known human pathogens are nonzoonotic—not transmissible from animals to humans—and the distinction between zoonotic and nonzoonotic infectious disease turns out not to be a bright line. For example, there are debates in the literature over whether foot-and-mouth disease is a zoonotic disease or not, and the recent history of avian influenza indicates that the difference between zoonotic and nonzoonotic can be a relatively small change in the viral genome. To avoid semantic difficulties, this chapter makes no distinction between nonzoonotic diseases (such as rinderpest) and infectious animal diseases that currently have a very low attack rate in people (such as highly pathogenic [H5N1] avian influenza, or HPAI). Similarly, the phrase "health and well-being" I use in the widest possible sense in this chapter to underscore the pervasive effects of animal disease in human populations.

Early Examples of the Consequences of a Nonzoonotic Disease

In 1792, an epidemic of a venereally transmitted disease broke out in horses kept in the studs and stables of Prussia.[1] It was a fatal disease that caused considerable damage to a large industry that employed many people. The disease spread throughout Europe and ultimately to North America. The disease was a dourine, a venereally transmitted trypanosomal infection of equids. The veterinarians and farm workers of the time knew that this disease was not transmissible to people, even to stable lads who had "excoriations" on their hands. But the disease alarmed them nevertheless. Horses were essential to nineteenth- and early twentieth-century economies. Before the steam engine, the horse and its relatives were the fastest and most reliable form of transport, and horses were crucial to warfare long after the development of firearms. The modern-day equivalent of the dourine pandemic would be the threat of a global oil shortage. The only counter to dourine was a nonpharmaceutical intervention (NPI)—the identification and isolation of affected animals.

The point of this two-hundred-year-old example is to show that globalization is not a recent phenomenon. Dourine was recognized in North Africa for centuries before it was recorded in Europe. Long-established channels of trade as well as European colonial expansion, which mixed missionary zeal with commercial interest and national prestige, brought the disease to Europe and, eventually, to North America. Admittedly, the pace of spread was slower than it would be today, but when a disease did arrive in a new location, there were few effective interventions in the veterinary armory, and almost all were NPIs.

The economic threat represented by infectious animal disease in the eighteenth and nineteenth centuries was well understood by veterinary professionals of the time. Indeed, the foreword to George Flemming's 1882 textbook, *Animal Plagues* (from which the dourine example was taken), makes it clear that one of Flemming's principal goals in writing the book was to make sure that the economic and social meaning of the catastrophic foot-and-mouth disease and rinderpest epidemics of the 1860s was not lost on the governments of the time. Infectious diseases in animals could not be ignored. These rumblings continued for fifty years, but it was the dramatic appearance of rinderpest in Belgium in

1920 and the subsequent international conference convened by the French in response that led to the founding of the OIE, now called the World Organisation for Animal Health. The OIE was explicitly international. It was founded to prevent devastating epidemics that could hamper world trade, and it was also recognized that the OIE had a role to play in improving public health.[2]

Similar organizations were also being created at a national level. For example, according to the published history of the Animal and Plant Health Inspection Service (APHIS) of the U.S. Department of Agriculture, the Bureau of Animal Industry, one of the several agencies that were later combined to form APHIS, was created mostly in response to the threat presented by contagious bovine pleuropneumonia. This disease was introduced into the United States in 1843. In 1879, the British government placed severe restrictions on the import of U.S. cattle and cattle products (*plus ça change...*), and in 1884 the United States created the Bureau of Animal Industry to eradicate the infection, which it did, in 1892— six years before the aerosol-transmitted mycoplasma (*Mycoplasma mycoides* subsp. *mycoides*) responsible for the disease was identified and cultured.

A Complacent Mind-Set

Until quite recently, Flemming's seminal book on animal plagues had been consigned to a box in a basement at the University of Pennsylvania, an action symptomatic of the mind-set that many scientists shared in those halcyon days when antibiotics worked, when new, safe, and effective antiparasitic drugs were appearing on the market with dependable frequency, and when mass vaccinations had reduced the occurrence of foot-and-mouth disease (for example) in Europe to such low levels that it was deemed less risky and certainly much cheaper to simply stop vaccinating—the days, that is, when pharmaceutical interventions seemed to have dealt infectious diseases in animals a telling blow. It was forgotten, or at least few chose to remember, that pharmaceutical interventions usually create a much more intense selection pressure than NPIs, and eventually, natural selection stepped in with a reminder that the respite was brief, and that even those of us living in the developed world should regard infectious diseases in animals from the same egocentric viewpoint as did those eighteenth and nineteenth century veterinarians and governments.

If anyone decides to write a new version of Flemming's book to cover the last 100 years, it can be conjectured, with some confidence, that the general historical arc will be something like this. Globalization was an established fact from the start of the twentieth century; animal infections had already been transported by colonial farmers to the far corners of the European empires. The common liver fluke, *Fasciola hepatica*, will serve as a typical example. This parasite is well established in Europe, North America, Australia, and New Zealand, as well as in parts of Asia, Africa, and South America. Prior to the 1960s, the safe control of fascioliosis depended mostly on NPIs (in short, farmers kept their sheep away from wet pastures, and various forecasting systems were developed to assist in that process). By the beginning of the 1970s there were several efficacious and very safe pharmaceutical interventions on the market, and they were heavily used, especially in places like Australia. Lately, drug resistance has severely impeded that control effort, and the ability to control this parasite as effectively as we did for a few short years is inexorably diminishing. We can find similar instances among the bacteria and viruses. For example, foot-and-mouth disease was introduced several times into North America early in the twentieth century. Its rate of spread was much slower than would be predicted in today's agricultural economy, which was just as well, because once again effective control depended on an NPI—isolation and depopulation. These strategies worked well because the rate of spread was slow and foot-and-mouth disease is an infection with a relatively small basic reproduction number. Collaborative surveillance and control agreements with countries to the south of the United States have succeeded in keeping the virus out of the United States for more than seventy years, and even on those continents that could not be quite so easily isolated from disease introductions, the advent of a vaccine in the middle of the century held out real promise that we could base trade agreements on the assumption that it would be possible for many countries to maintain a virus-free state for considerable periods of time. Today, of course, the projected and actual rate of spread of the foot-and-mouth disease virus in the developed agricultural nations are much greater than in earlier times, and many countries have relinquished pharmaceutical interventions that still work out of fear of jeopardizing their trading status.

The Rinderpest Pandemic

We find ourselves in a phase in which pharmaceutical interventions are beginning to fail, the rate of geographic spread of animal disease is dismayingly rapid, and current trade agreements render us unwilling to return to control strategies that we know work—at least for a time. In short, we are having to learn all over again why we should never be sanguine about infectious diseases in domestic animals. However, the problem should not be overstated. In the context of emerging and reemerging disease, there is a tendency to resort to the language of catastrophe. For example, the rinderpest epidemic of the late nineteenth century (1896–1898) is repeatedly alluded to as a typical example of what a nonzoonotic disease can do to the economic and social fabric of a country. Summaries of the damage done by the disease in Basutoland and elsewhere in southern Africa make sober reading.[3] Rinderpest killed more than 95 percent of African herds throughout southern Africa. It threatened to provoke an unprecedented rural crisis: it killed milk-producing cows, depriving people—especially growing babies—of essential dietary requirements, and, in wiping out the plow-drawing oxen, it destroyed the means of agricultural production and precipitated a food crisis. By killing cattle, rinderpest threatened to wipe out the only capital of the people and to restrict future capital. The epidemic was compounded by a series of droughts and it ended just as the Boer War started, with disease, famine, social fragmentation, changes in migration and settlement patterns. . . . It's all very familiar, and there is no doubt that it is all true. Indeed, the threat to sustainable livelihoods presented by epidemic animal disease in pastoral settings is much the same today as it was in 1897. But it is an ill wind that blows nobody good. The consequences of epidemics like the rinderpest epidemic turn out to be rather subtle. Their severity depends on the kinds of coping strategies that the people involved are able to employ. In this particular case, the Basotho who lost their animals turned a potential famine into a food shortage by reverting to high-intensity agriculture using the hoe rather that the plow. In addition, the reduction of the bovine population through rinderpest decreased the pressure on available grazing, enabling previously overgrazed pastures to recover. In Basutoland, at least, the rinderpest outbreak was a temporary setback, and some actually profited by it. With cattle dead, the demand for mutton put a high premium on slaughter sheep. The South African War, in 1899, created an insatiable labor market and offered the Basotho a temporary opportunity to cushion the effects of the epidemic and get cash to restock.

We see this "ill wind phenomenon" quite frequently. The foot-and-mouth disease epidemic in Taiwan in 1996–1997 put an end to its lucrative export trade in pigs to Japan. It seems likely that the Taiwanese will not reclaim that market, at least in the short term, because the demand for pork in Japan was satisfied by an increase in exports from the United States and Canada, which still retain that market. When bovine spongiform encephalitis (BSE) was discovered in older cattle in Canada and the United States, more than fifty countries suspended imports of North American ruminants and ruminant products—and the United States closed the Canadian border to cattle movement. This was a disaster for Canada, which had previously exported a large quantity of its beef to the United States. The United States, on the other hand, was left relatively unaffected. Because the border with Canada had closed, there was a shortage of imported beef, so U.S. beef prices increased. Not everybody necessarily suffers, or suffers in the same way.

The Modern-Day Consequences of Large-Scale Epidemic Disease in Animals

Failure to adequately control large-scale epidemic disease in animals has multiple consequences. There are direct economic losses;

indirect multiplier effects (on agriculture-related industries, trade, or tourism); multiple opportunities for fraud and other criminal acts; and logistical, environmental, social, and political difficulties associated with the disposal of carcasses. There is usually controversy concerning control methods and a concomitant loss of confidence in government. Public anxiety about the risk of human disease increases, even with respect to nonzoonotic diseases, and there may be damaging academic controversy.

The direct and indirect economic effects of epidemics in animal populations are well documented. I conclude with some examples of the consequences of animal epidemics that receive less attention but are nevertheless valid indices of the adverse effects of such epidemics on the health and well-being of people. One unexpected consequence is the greater opportunity such epidemics present for criminal activity. Only a few cases of BSE have been reported in animals in Japan, but the Japanese response has been strenuous. Beef was removed from sale for a period, and wholesalers were compensated to make sure compliance was as good as it could be—but this presented opportunities for the unscrupulous. The Japanese Snow Brand Food Company admitted repackaging Australian beef as Japanese so as to claim government compensation. In Britain, farms left deserted following depopulation in response to the 2001 foot-and-mouth disease epidemic were easy targets for thieves. During the course of the epidemic, disinfectant barrels were stolen more frequently than any other item. Later, thieves turned their attention to larger equipment, such as tractors. During that same epidemic, the ban on animal movement was regularly flouted, and there were multiple claims that the compensation system was being abused. Four years later, on the other side of the world, exploiting the fear that British foot-and-mouth disease engendered, a letter was sent to the New Zealand government stating that the foot-and-mouth disease virus had been released on Waiheke Island. The letter contained demands for money and changes to the tax system. Movement controls were immediately instituted, every farm was inspected every forty-eight hours, and there was an intensive trace-back of animals and at-risk goods exported off the island. A second letter claimed the first was a hoax, but it was a very expensive hoax.

The final tally was in excess of NZ $200 million. More recently, in the midst of an epidemic of H5N1 avian influenza, Zainal Baharuddin, the Inspector General of the Indonesian Agriculture Ministry, released a statement to the press in which it was reported that local producers, with the collusion of some ministry officials, had intentionally lowered the quality of avian influenza vaccine to make more profit from the government contract. The urge to profit from the misfortune of others has always been with us. Those Basotho who experienced the rinderpest epidemic over a hundred years ago didn't just sit back passively and let it happen to them. Some tried to restock by raiding Boer cattle herds just over the border, and some rather duplicitously arranged to look after Boer herds until the Boer War was over. Basutoland was a British protectorate at the time, and from the British point of view this was undoubtedly treason. Because very few herds were returned to the Boers when the war ended, this was, from the Boer point of view, straightforward theft.

Before leaving the topic of criminality, it should be noted that animal disease epidemics can be the *result* of criminal activity as well as a precipitating factor. Once of the most obvious examples is the introduction of the foot-and-mouth disease virus into a population of pigs in northern England via illegally imported meat. In fact, the extent and frequency with which national borders are assaulted and crossed by pathogens concealed in animals and plants—or in animal and plant products—are simply astonishing. In the United States, the employee newsletter of the Customs and Border Protection Agency noted that on a typical day, the agency seizes 1,145 prohibited meat and plant materials (including 147 agricultural pests). Among the seized materials are smuggled birds, a particularly sensitive topic in today's world of exotic Newcastle disease and highly pathogenic avian influenza. The average number of birds estimated to be smuggled into the United States each year is in the tens of thousands. The USDA Web site suggests that smuggling birds is the second most profitable smuggling operation across U.S. borders.

Animal epidemics are also a source of serious social and political tension. Depopulation, an NPI, is still the method of choice for controlling many infectious diseases of livestock, even those for which pharmaceutical interventions could be substituted. It is an effective and rapid solution to the problem. It also appeals to those sectors whose definition of success is the resumption of trade as quickly as possible. There is no denying, though, that the destruction of hundreds, thousands, and sometimes millions of uninfected animals as a disease control strategy is an ugly process, and it is certainly an unpopular strategy with the general public, especially when the scale of depopulation is so great that the people cannot help but notice. For some, the apparently disproportionate number of uninfected animals killed is simply offensive because it does not seem necessary. For others, it is an ethical or esthetic issue, and confusion and misunderstanding abut the decisions with respect to which animals are killed and why add to the general distaste—especially if there appear to be available pharmaceutical interventions that might have been used instead. Mix in concerns (some well-founded, others less so) about the possibility of environmental pollution, and you have the basis for social unrest. A classic instance of this was the response to foot-and-mouth disease in Mexico by the U.S. and Mexican governments,[4] which entailed depopulating animals in infected regions. Poor rural Mexicans reacted to this solution with drastic and sometimes violent protests. The leaders of both nations began to fear broad unrest and to worry that conflict would endanger security, trade, investment, and even the stability of a postwar world thought to be threatened by communism. Within a year, Mexican and American leadership had changed tactics and begun to vaccinate the infected center of the country, over intense U.S. industry opposition. Just as dramatically, four months into the foot-and-mouth disease outbreak in Britain in 2001, public impatience and anger were so great that the government ministry responsible for animal health was abolished and replaced by a mere department sequestered within some other ministry. The same epidemic engendered a poisonous argument between some government veterinarians and several of the groups responsible for the mathematical models that informed government policy.

Even when an animal infection is not zoonotic, a large-scale epidemic can have severe consequences for human health in the strictest sense. For example, the status of foot-and-mouth disease as a zoonotic disease is still debated. Even if it is, the attack rate in people is very, very small. For several years, however, there have been anecdotal reports of severe psychological illness among the farmers whose herds were depopulated during the 2001 epidemic. A recent case-control study of Dutch farmers suggests that the anecdotes may well be true. The proportion of farmers with signs of posttraumatic stress syndrome was greater among those whose herds were depopulated than among those whose herds were unaffected.[5]

There are other ways, too, in which human health can be directly affected by animal diseases that are not in themselves a particular threat to human health. Another Dutch study, this one looking at the aftermath of the 2001–2002 HPAI outbreak, found an unanticipated 50 percent increase in the number of cases of *Salmonella* infections in people. This was attributed to an increase in the importation of *Salmonella*-contaminated eggs. The increased imports were necessary to make up for the shortfall created by depopulating domestic poultry flocks.[6]

Conclusion

The consequences of infectious diseases in domestic animal populations are multiple, pervasive, and often subtle—not everyone suffers, for example. Nor is it only zoonotic infections that can affect human health and well-being. If human health and well-being are understood to include the integrity of the social, economic, and political frameworks that we depend on for stability and security, then animal epidemics can represent a serious threat indeed.

References

1. G. Fleming (1882), *Animal Plagues*, vol. 2 (London: Balliere, Tindal and Cox).

2. M. Teissier (2006), "A Brief History of the World Organization for Animal Health," presented at the Tenth European Conference of Medical and Health Libraries, Cluj-Napoca, Romania, September 11–16.

3. P. Phoofolo (2003), "Face to Face with Famine: The BaSotho and the Rinderpest, 1897–1899," *Journal of Southern African Studies* 29, no. 2 (June).

4. H. Johnson (1951), "Foot-and-Mouth Disease Campaign in Mexico," *Veterinary Medicine* 46: 5.

5. M. Olff, M. W. J. Koetter, E. H. Van Haaften, P. H. Kersten, and B. P. R. Gersons (2005), "Impact of a Foot and Mouth Disease Crisis on Post-Traumatic Stress Symptoms in Farmers," *British Journal of Psychiatry* 186: 165–66.

6. W. van Pelt, D. Mevius, H. G. Stoelhorst, S. Kovats, A. W. van de Giessen, W. Wannet, and Y. T. H. P. Duynhoven (2004), "A Large Increase of *Salmonella* Infections in 2003 in The Netherlands: Hot Summer or Side Effect of the Avian Influenza Outbreak?" *Euro Surveillance* 9: 17–19.

Part II
The Food Industry

Chapter 7
The Global Food Industry
David Harlan and Candace Jacobs

This chapter provides an introduction to the global food industry through the example and experiences of two international companies, Cargill and H-E-B Grocery Company. Cargill is an international provider of food, agricultural, and risk management products and services. It has 153,000 employees in sixty-six countries and is engaged in the global meat trade. H-E-B Grocery Company is one of the largest independently owned food retailers in the United States. It has over 300 stores and 56,000 employees in Texas and Mexico.

An Overview of Cargill

Cargill produces and distributes crop nutrients and feed ingredients to farmers and beef, dairy, pork, and poultry producers and animal feeders. It originates and processes grain, oilseeds, and other agricultural commodities for distribution to makers of food, feed, and other products. It provides vegetable oil, salt, and starch products and services, industrial applications for agricultural products, and steel products and services. Cargill is also a proprietary investor, alternative asset manager, and provider of risk management products and services. To take just a few examples of the global nature of the Cargill business, the company has poultry production and processing businesses in North America, Central America, South America, Asia, and Europe. It has beef operations in Australia, the United States, Canada, and Argentina, and pork operations in Brazil and the United States. It has egg-processing plants in Europe, the United States, and Canada. This U.S.-based company now has more employees outside the United States than inside. Its stated vision and goal is to be the global leader in nourishing people. The company states that access to food is a basic human right and that everyone in the world has that right. Food is for nourishment, it should never be used as a political weapon. It agrees with the World Health Organization (WHO) and others that global poverty and hunger are the major public health challenge we face today. It sees economic growth as the engine for alleviating poverty and hunger worldwide. It is Cargill's belief that trade promotes economic growth; it reduces poverty and improves nourishment, and therefore improves public health.

About 400 million metric tons of animal proteins are consumed globally, about half by people in Asia. One benefit is that the global meat trade allows companies like Cargill to produce the required proteins in areas of the world that are best suited to production. It also permits and promotes the creation of specialized production systems (just eggs, or seafood, or beef, or chicken) and allows companies to compensate for production variations around the world. If one country or region of the world has a particularly good harvest or a particularly poor harvest, another area of the world can make up the deficit or take the surplus production. Companies like Cargill see global trade as a way to optimize the value of parts. For example, how many people eat liver or intestine on a regular basis? Neither of these products is popular in North America, and they therefore constitute a surplus that can be traded to other areas of the world, where they may be more valuable. Global trade can also assist developing countries by compensating for deficits in local resources. For example, some major population centers, such as China and India, have insufficient freshwater to permit the long-term production of feed grains for livestock. Global trade means that the grain, for example, can be produced elsewhere in the world and shipped to areas where production at the required level is not possible, or animals can be raised elsewhere and animal products shipped to areas in need. For example, the United States and Brazil are both major exporters of poultry meat because, in both countries, there is an abundance of the required grain and water. Similarly, South America, Australia, and Canada all have sufficient land mass to graze cattle and to produce a surplus of beef, which is then shipped globally.

Disease Is the Major Challenge Faced by the Global Meat Trade

A major challenge to the global meat trade is disease. Disease is a critical issue that needs to be managed in order to maintain global supply chains of meat. For a company like Cargill that manages international supply chains from origination (farm) to destination (food companies and quick service restaurants), the erection of nontariff trade barriers can lead to severe disruption. The recent confluence of animal diseases such as bovine spongiform encephalopathy (BSE), foot-and-mouth disease, and highly pathogenic (H5N1) avian influenza (HPAI) has alerted the food industry to the importance of risk management as a vital element in disease control. It is increasingly appreciated that many disease control programs do not require a complete suspension of trade to be effective, and also that it may not be possible to remain completely free of disease, import bans notwithstanding. The current outbreak of H5N1 avian influenza in Asia provides a good example. Even in the face of such an outbreak, international standards indicate that certain products, such as cooked poultry meat, can be safely traded even in the unlikely event that they came from infected animals. It is also possible to raise birds in a disease-free way in countries or regions where H5N1 avian influenza persists, and companies like Cargill do just that. In the past, there was little trust between the food industry and other stakeholders in global food systems (such as OIE, the World Bank, WHO, intergovernmental agencies, and universities), and, although there was some limited communication back and forth among these various stakeholders, there were clear differences in priorities. However, one consequence of the H5N1 avian influenza in Asia and elsewhere has been to persuade all the stakeholders that they have many shared interests and that deficiencies in the capacity to control animal disease undercut trade and reduce the rate of economic development, especially in the developing world. Furthermore, it is now understood that failure to implement global, science-based trade standards has a huge impact on our ability to use risk management strategies to deal with animal disease. In the past, many stakeholders, the food industry especially, failed to recognize the public global good of animal and human public health systems. That is starting to change. Formerly adversarial relationships are transmuting into partnerships, including public-private partnerships, in which all the stakeholders share the risk and responsibility. Companies like Cargill are promoting the linkages among animal health, public health, and food safety, and these linkages collectively leverage the strengths of each stakeholder.

An example of this kind of collaboration is the "One World, One Health" program promoted by the Wildlife Conservation Society. As a result of that program, Cargill and other food industry companies, in partnership with the OIE, the World Bank, and the Food and Agriculture Organization, created SSAFE (an acronym for Safe Supply of Affordable Food Everywhere), whose object is to provide a safe harbor for dialogue between and among the food industry, NGOs, and intergovernmental agencies. The goals are to leverage resources, to advocate harmonized trading policies, to work together to support an uninterrupted sustainable food supply for all countries, to protect human and animal health, and to help nations improve their veterinary and public health infrastructure. A first step has been to create a workable compartmentalization model through which biocontainment can help keep subpopulations of animals free of disease, regardless of what diseases may persist in other parts of the region or country. The intention is that trade with protected compartments within a country could be maintained regardless of the disease status of the country as a whole. The difference between compartmentalization and "zoning" (an OIE term referring to the designation of particular areas of a country as disease-free) is that the compartments need not represent specific geographic regions. The idea of a compartment is that it is a biosecure entity. An integrated poultry system (hatchery, processor, breeders, feed mill, processing plant, rendering plant) distributed over several regions might constitute a compartment because it is integrated and not connected with other domestic poultry (such as found in backyard farms) or even with other integrators. Compartments may cross regions, but trade would continue to flow within and out of that compartment even if there is disease in one or more of the regions containing the compartment.

An Overview of H-E-B Grocery Company

H-E-B was started in 1905 in Kerrville, Texas. The company has about 300 stores and serves South and Central Texas and northern Mexico. It is the thirteenth largest grocery in the United States, with more than $13 billion in annual sales. The company manages five major U.S. distribution complexes and eleven manufacturing plants, and promotes a corporate culture of helping neighbors in need (more than 5 percent of H-E-B's pretax earnings goes to civic and charitable organizations). There are four store formats: the familiar general food and drug store; a "plus format," which is a big box store that sells furniture and related items; an upscale "Central Market"; and the new "Mi Tienda" format, aimed at the Latino market in the United States. H-E-B operations in Mexico began in 1997. There are twenty-six stores in different cities, and a distribution center in Monterrey. A new distribution center in Weslaco, Texas, serves stores in both Texas and Mexico. H-E-B's main competition in Mexico is from Wal-Mart, Soriana, and Hegante.

Supermarkets dominate the way food is handled globally and have an impact on the way food is produced in developing countries, and American-style supermarkets are increasing standards for food safety, animal welfare, and environmental protection globally.

In the United States, over the past sixty years, the growth in the grocery business was spurred by the growth in supportive infrastructure. For example, the development of the interstate highway system and the introduction of refrigerated trucks meant that suppliers no longer had to use railroads. This permitted deliveries beyond the central market districts. The rise of distribution centers allowed better supply chain management (through technology such as cold chain maintenance and delivery), and thus supermarket companies could manage their own quality. The introduction of standardized crates, cartons, standard-sized pallets, and unitization has made moving things around much easier. When supermarkets can manage their own supply chain through vertical integration they can save at least 10 percent on delivery and labor costs, which is a large amount in a penny business like the grocery business. Worldwide, the more recent pattern in supermarket development has been chain consolidation, with most larger entities benchmarking against Wal-Mart. Wal-Mart has 6,447 outlets worldwide, most of them outside the United States.

In Mexico, where H-E-B is increasing the number of its stores, supermarket development over the past ten to twenty years has been very rapid indeed. Nevertheless, there are still deficits in the supply chain. The good road networks in Mexico tend to be between the bedroom communities and the large metropolitan centers; the road network in rural areas is less well developed. The goal, of course, is a fully integrated truck and rail network by which high-quality food could be delivered in a consistent, cost-effective manner. Harmonization of product standards is still a huge problem in Mexico. Existing public standards deal primarily with sanitary and phytosanitary standards, not food safety per se.

Issues to Consider When Moving a Grocery Business into Another Country

The North American Free Trade Agreement (NAFTA) and its two supplements, the North American Agreement on Environmental Cooperation (NAAEC) and the North American Agreement on Labor Cooperation (NAALC), went into effect on January 1, 1994, and have been extremely useful for companies and businesses in the United States interested in expanding operations into Canada and Mexico (especially with respect to reducing tariffs and providing a vehicle for dispute resolution). But it is also important for such companies to know the national culture of the country they are proposing to enter. Local legislation dealing with labor issues, planning and zoning, and regulations that affect opening hours can make a big difference in whether or not the new business will be successful. Decisions also have to be made regarding whether the business will make global or local purchases of the items it sells. It appears to make sense to purchase locally because this reduces transportation costs, but how can companies then get the required quality produce, at the required cost, on a routine basis?

One of the biggest challenges H-E-B faced when it was procuring supplies in Mexico from Mexican firms was the absence of well-defined quality standards. There was poor supply chain management, and the physical infrastructure was inadequate. One solution was to increase the volume of fresh fruit and vegetable shipments purchased from small to medium-sized Mexican growers (this focus on smaller producers was consistent with the H-E-B philosophy with respect social responsibility—to develop close ties with small to medium-sized producers and to assist them in transforming their production and business practices). In parallel with this emphasis on smaller producers, H-E-B, in partnership with the Mexico Agriculture Ministry, developed the Suppliers Development Program at the Tecnológico de Monterrey, a private Mexican educational institution founded in 1943 that has academic centers in Mexico and other Latin American countries. Any supplier who wishes to supply goods to the H-E-B stores in Mexico must go through this two-day program. The program educates suppliers on the quality assurance standards H-E-B requires its suppliers to know and to adopt, and H-E-B will sometimes offset the cost of attending this program if those who attend and become certified eventually do business with H-E-B. The partnership with Tecnológico de Monterrey was recently expanded to include a program on HACCP procedures for improving food safety. Interestingly, food safety in the H-E-B stores in Mexico is the same as or better than food safety in U.S. stores. Labor in Mexico is cheaper than in the United States, so the company can pay more people to clean the floors, walls, and ceilings. Not only does this contribute to improved food safety, it encourages shoppers to come through.

Businesses also need to think about how they will enter a chosen country. There are three different ways: by joint venture (the Wal-Mart strategy), acquisition (buy something that is already there), or build your own (organic growth). Joint venture methods provide quick access to local markets and good expertise locally, and sometimes the advantage of being perceived as a local company. The advantages of the build-your-own (organic growth) model are flexibility and freedom of choice of choice with respect to store location.

Merchandising strategies must also be considered. In Mexico, H-E-B merchandising strategies have to be evaluated in the light of what happens in the traditional open air markets. For example, public markets apply different prices for the same commodity. They charge a premium for the highest quality produce for any given commodity. Supermarkets, on the other hand, charge the same price for the same commodity of a particular size, regardless of its maturity or cosmetic appearance, and supermarkets have more formal oversight of weights and measures issues than do public markets. Furthermore, pricing strategies that might work in the United States will not necessarily work in a less developed country like Mexico. Strategies such as the "buy two and get the third free" ploy familiar to U.S. shoppers do not work in countries where shoppers cannot afford to purchase two items, or in places where transporting large numbers of items is difficult or perishable items cannot be safely stored in homes. Clearly, merchandising strategies need to take into account the characteristics of those who shop. Mexican shoppers shop about three times as often as U.S. shoppers do. Shoppers in the United States get into stores 2.2 times a week on average; Mexican shoppers shop more than once a day. One of the reasons is that Mexican shoppers have more limited access to automobiles: shoppers who walk home or take public transportation to households that have limited household refrigeration capacity do not carry much. Accordingly, customers prefer to purchase fresh ripe produce and fresh ready-to-eat foods or foods they can prepare for consumption that day. As a consequence, product selection becomes more important. Global companies are able to import products from the cheapest sources and so can offer a broader selection of items for sale than the traditional public markets. But variety or even quality may not necessarily be what the consumer is looking for. Mexican consumers, for example, want food fresh—fruit salads, fresh cut products, packaged green salads —and they want to eat it today. Freshness is something supermarkets can achieve because they can maintain a cold chain from the site of origin until the produce is placed on the shelves. This is something general markets find difficult. The general markets are often less safe for shoppers in countries like Mexico. Personal safety is an important issue in Mexico, especially for some of the higher income households. The bright lights, wide aisles, and security guards that supermarkets can provide are real inducements to shop, compared with the conditions of the darker and more crowded traditional market. Supermarkets also have superior climate control for perishable products, and they have superior climate control for their customers.

Conclusion

Both Cargill and H-E-B have found it advantageous to engage in public-private partnerships: partnerships between commercial enterprises, academic institutions, and government agencies (among others). The partnerships extend across national boundaries. This is consistent with the vision and social values of both companies, but it has a straightforward commercial rationale, too. The partnerships promote and improve animal health and the consistency and safety of the food supply and are an important tool in creating and expanding trading relationships, but they also are fundamental to the global maintenance of human health and well-being.

Chapter 8
Farming the Sea
The Revolution in Aquaculture

Richard Langan

Population growth, as well as greater consumer preference, has resulted in a growing demand for seafood, a trend that is projected to continue into the future.[1] Production from capture fisheries, the primary source of seafood just two decades ago, has leveled off and by most projections will remain stagnant or decline, depending on management and regulatory measures implemented by fishing nations.[2,3] In contrast, aquaculture production has increased by approximately 10 percent per year since 1980 and has played an important role in filling the gap between seafood supply and demand. The most recent data indicate that aquaculture now supplies nearly 50 percent of the seafood consumed by humans.[1] While aquaculture production is projected to continue to increase, growth will not keep pace with demand, owing to political, environmental, economic, and resource constraints on the growth of land-based and nearshore marine culture, and the gap between supply and demand is projected to reach 40 million metric tons by 2030. This ever-increasing divide is particularly critical for the United States, where aquaculture development lags far behind the rest of the world and imports constitute 70 percent of the seafood consumed. If the United States does not find a way to increase aquaculture production, American consumers will soon be confronted with higher prices and decreased availability of seafood. Farming in offshore marine waters has been identified as one potential option for increased production; however, wind and wave conditions in most of the world's oceans pose significant technical and operational challenges. Offshore waters require a completely new engineering approach since equipment and methods currently used for fish and shellfish production in protected nearshore waters are unsuitable for the open ocean. Despite these challenges, there is sufficient rationale for pursuing the development of open ocean farming. Favorable features of open ocean waters, such as ample space, tremendous carry capacity, the potential to reduce some of the negative environmental impacts of coastal fish farming, and optimal environmental conditions for a wide variety of marine species, have encouraged many countries, including the United States, to consider offshore development.

The Approach

Interest in farming in offshore waters in the United States has largely been driven by academic institutions in partnership with private industry, and by federal government initiatives in response to the need for greater domestic self-sufficiency in seafood supply. Through competitive research programs and congressionally directed funding initiated in the late 1990s, the Department of Commerce's National Oceanic and Atmospheric Administration (NOAA) was instrumental in supporting offshore aquaculture development. Targeting husbandry methods for new marine species, advanced engineering technologies, and the development of environmentally responsible practices, NOAA made some strategic investments in regional R&D programs in New Hampshire, Hawaii, and Puerto Rico. The New Hampshire project, led by a multidisciplinary team from the University of New Hampshire (UNH), best illustrates the U.S. approach to the design, development, and assessment of offshore farming systems.

Encouraged by promising results from a number of small-scale engineering projects and hatchery research on the production of cold-water species in the mid-1990s, UNH initiated the Open Ocean Aquaculture Project in 1998. The goal of the project is to stimulate the development of an environmentally sustainable off-shore aquaculture industry, thereby increasing seafood production, creating new employment opportunities, and contributing to regional and national economic and community development. With funding from NOAA and in partnership with local fishing cooperatives and a commercial marine fish hatchery, and with the collaboration of several regional research institutions, UNH established an offshore aquaculture R&D facility in the Gulf of Maine in 1999. The offshore platform, located six miles off the New Hampshire coastline in 185 feet of water and fully exposed to the extreme conditions of the Northwest Atlantic, is approved by state and federal regulatory authorities for multispecies commercial production. The project team has focused on coordinated research efforts in the development of engineering design and assessment tools; the deployment and evaluation of engineered systems, including moorings, cages, feeders, and remote observation and operations systems; the development of rearing techniques for a number of native marine species; and implementation of management practices to mitigate the potential environmental impacts of fish farming. Engineered systems at the site consist of a submerged grid mooring system that can accommodate four submersible cages for finfish culture, two submerged longlines for suspended molluscan shellfish culture, and surface structures that include remotely operated feeders, acoustic biotelemetry systems, and oceanographic instrumentation. Fish species cultured at the site include summer flounder (*Paralichthyus dentatus*), Atlantic halibut (*Hippoglossus hippoglossus*), haddock (*Melanogrammus aeglefinis*), and Atlantic cod (*Gadus morhua*). In addition, blue mussels (*Mytilus edulis*) and Atlantic sea scallops (*Placopecten magellanicus*) have been grown on submerged longlines adjacent to the fish cages.

Environmental concerns have been addressed by the implementation of management practices designed to minimize potential impacts and a rigorous environmental monitoring program to measure any changes to the surrounding environment. To address escapes, the project has developed a suite of engineering tools to design and evaluate mooring systems and cages that can withstand extreme environmental conditions and avoid catastrophic losses due to storm damage. Cages are submerged 12 to 15 m below the sea surface to reduce the risk of ship collisions. A containment management plan, based on the principles of a HACCP risk analysis program, includes frequent inspection and maintenance, as well as procedures to prevent escapement during stocking, sampling, harvesting, and transport operations. All fish cultured at the site are native to the area, and to date, all juveniles stocked in the sea cages have been the offspring of wild parents. Therefore, any escapees would be genetically identical to local stocks. Waste feed is managed by the use of remote, real-time video monitoring and control of feeding operations, so that feed delivery can be stopped when the fish are satiated. The adjacent culture of extractive species such as mussels and scallops is used to balance the inputs of nitrogen and phosphorus resulting from the addition of feed for fish. Fish health is managed using vaccination prior to stocking and by maintaining optimal environmental conditions, such as appropriate temperature and dissolved oxygen concentration, to minimize stress. Dead or moribund fish are removed promptly to reduce the risk of reservoirs of pathogens developing as a result of decomposition. To date, no antibiotics or parasite treatments have been administered.

An initial site assessment conducted in 1998 established a baseline of seafloor, oceanographic, and environmental conditions.[4] Numerical models were used to predict the dispersion and deposition of particulates and dissolved constituents, and twenty monitoring stations were established to represent impact, mixing, far field, and distant far field zones. The stations are monitored periodically to detect any changes in benthic community characteristics and sediment and water chemistry that may be attributed to farming operations.

Projects in Hawaii and Puerto Rico have taken an approach to the UNH initiative, employing submersible cages in offshore sites, culturing fish native to the region, implementing best management practices, and monitoring environmental effects. The species selected for culture include Pacific threadfin (*Polydactylus sexfilis*) in Oahu, amberjack (*Seriola rivoliana*) off the Kona coast of the Big Island, and cobia (*Rachycentron canadum*) at the farm located off the coast of Culebra Island in Puerto Rico.

Collectively, these regional projects have been successful in demonstrating that finfish and shellfish culture systems can be installed, maintained, and operated in the harshest oceanic conditions. Growth performance, feed conversion, and health of the culture species at all locations have been excellent, indicating that the open ocean environment may provide some advantages over nearshore or land-based culture systems.[5-7] The results of environmental monitoring at the sites have shown little or no change in environmental conditions, indicating that with properly sited farms, appropriate system design, and sound management and husbandry practices, the environmental impacts of offshore finfish culture are negligible.[1,8,9] Each of the projects has led to private sector activity, with commercial fish farms operating in Hawaii and Puerto Rico and commercial mussel culture under way off the coast of New Hampshire.

Conclusion

Pilot projects in the United States have demonstrated that open ocean aquaculture is feasible and can be conducted in an environmentally responsible manner; however, a number of technical and operational challenges have been identified that must be addressed in order to achieve the high levels of production needed to fill the projected gap between seafood supply and demand. Additional R&D should focus on the design and anchoring of surface structures such as feeders and monitoring systems, the development of highly mechanized and fully integrated systems to achieve greater efficiency and ensure worker safety, more precise depth control and alternative materials for cages, and the use of alternative energy sources such as wind, waves, and currents to power farming equipment. Biological research should be directed toward domestication of new species to regulate the spawning period, improve egg and larval quality, enhance growth rates, and delay sexual maturation. Research is also needed to develop optimal diets and to identify alternative protein and lipid sources, to reduce dependency on fishmeal and fish oil as feed ingredients. In addition, for many marine species under development, very little is known about potential diseases or parasites, so close attention must be paid to fish health issues as culture of these species expands. The technical challenges for the large-scale development of open ocean farming are not insignificant; however, based on the advances that have occurred over a relatively short period, the goals are achievable, provided an adequate and sustained investment of public funds is made in R&D. In the United States, social and political resistance to aquaculture development is probably the greatest impediment to the large-scale development of offshore farming.

It is widely acknowledged that future increases in seafood production will likely come from farming, not fishing. The growth of land-based and nearshore marine aquaculture in many developed countries, including the United States, is constrained by space, economics, and environmental concerns. For aquaculture to expand, the potential of farming offshore ocean waters must be explored. Over the past decade, there has been worldwide interest in exploring the potential for offshore production, and the United States has emerged as one of the leaders in developing and demonstrating technologies for open ocean culture. Offshore research and development projects in New Hampshire, Hawaii, and Puerto Rico have led to small-scale commercial production of finfish and shellfish, demonstrating that open ocean culture is indeed feasible and has great potential for future expansion. Despite the evidence that offshore farming is possible, a number of technical, economic, and political challenges must be addressed before large-scale production can be realized. Offshore aquaculture will be a technology-driven enterprise; therefore, continued investment in R&D is needed to achieve the level of efficiency required for economic viability. For development to occur in the United States, a sea change in social and political will must occur to allow the development of a business climate that will attract private sector investment in domestic operations. Otherwise, technology developed in the United States will be implemented overseas, and the United States will continue to experience the uncertain supply and high cost of imported seafood.

References

1. Food and Agriculture Organization (2006), State of World Aquaculture: 2006, FAO Fisheries Technical Paper 500 (Rome: FAO).

2. National Aeronautics and Oceanic Administration (2005), Fisheries of the United States—2003 (Washington, D.C.: NOAA), http://www.st.nmfs.gov/st1/fus/fus03/index.html.

3. B. Worm, E. B. Barbier, N. Beaumont, J. E. Duffy, C. Folke, B. S. Halpern, J. B. C. Jackson, H. K. Lotze, F. Micheli, S. R. Palumbi, E. Sala, E. K. Selkoe, J. J. Stachowicz, and R. Watson (2006), "Impacts of Biodiversity Loss on Ocean Ecosystem Services," *Science* 314: 787–90.

4. R. Grizzle, L. G. Ward, R. Langan, G. Schnaittacher, J. Dijkstra, and J. R. Adams (2003), "Environmental Monitoring at an Open Ocean Aquaculture Site in the Gulf of Maine: Results for 1997–2000," in *Open Ocean Aquaculture: From Research to Commercial Reality*, ed. C. J. Bridger and B. A. Costa-Pierce (Baton Rouge, La.: World Aquaculture Society), 105–19.

5. A. C. Ostrowski and C. E. Helsley (2003), "The Hawaii Offshore Aquaculture Research Project: Critical Research and Development Issues for Commercialization," in *Open Ocean Aquaculture: From Research to Commercial Reality*, ed. C. J. Bridger and B. A. Costa-Pierce (Baton Rouge, La.: World Aquaculture Society), 119–28.

6. W. H. Howell, W. H. Watson, and M. D. Chambers (2006), Offshore Production of Cod, Haddock and Halibut, CINEMar/Open Ocean Aquaculture Annual Progress Report for the Period from 1/01/05 to 12/31/05, Final Report for NOAA Grant No. NA16RP1718, Interim Progress Report for NOAA Grant No. NA04OAR4600155, submitted January 23, http://ooa.unh.edu.

7. D. Benetti, B. O'Hanlon, L. Brand, R. Orhun, I. Zink, P. Doulliet, J. Collins, C. Maxey, A. Danylchuk, D. Alston, and A. Cabarcas (2006), "Hatchery: On Growing Technology and Environmental Monitoring of Open Ocean Aquaculture of Cobia (*Rachycentron canadum*) in the Caribbean," World Aquaculture Society, abstract, in *Proceedings of Aquaculture 2006*, Florence, Italy, http://www.was.org/meetings/AbstractData.asp?AbstractId=10424.

8. C. E. Helsley and J. K. Kim (2005), "Mixing Downstream of a Submerged Fish Cage: A Numerical Study," *IEEE Journal of Oceanic Engineering* 30, no. 1: 12–19.

9. L. G. Ward, R. E. Grizzle, and J. D. Irish (2006), UNH OOA Environmental Monitoring Program, 2005, CINEMar/Open Ocean Aquaculture Annual Progress Report for the Period from 1/01/05 to 12/31/05, Final Report for NOAA Grant No. NA16RP1718, Interim Progress Report for NOAA Grant No. NA04OAR4600155, submitted January 23, http://ooa.unh.edu.

Chapter 9
Creating Risk
Antibiotic Resistance
Shelley Rankin

The incidence of antibiotic resistance is increasing worldwide. It is an emotional topic that is complicated by inadequate data and a natural tendency to resort to back-of-the-envelope calculations in defense of tenuous positions. This chapter sets out the basic issues and draws attention to some particular problems in the developing world. I offer no conclusions about causation.

Background

A 1996 World Health Organization (WHO) report stated that "A major cause of the antibiotic crisis is the uncontrolled and inappropriate use of antibiotics globally. They are used by too many people to treat the wrong kind of infections at the wrong dosage and for the wrong period of time."[1] The report went on to say, "Antibiotics and other antimicrobial agents are used in enormous amounts worldwide for the production of animal meat for human consumption. Some 170 billion tons of animal meat is produced every year. Drug resistant bacteria and other microbes are passed through the food chain to the consumer, where they may cause disease, or transfer the resistance to human pathogens." Antibiotic use in livestock is of premier importance, given the globalization of our food supply. Policies and guidelines have been developed worldwide on the containment of antibiotic resistance, and one of the biggest issues continues to be the use of antibiotics in livestock production. "Meat producers have fed growth-promoting antibiotics to food animals for years. Recently, scientists have raised concerns that, in conjunction with the general overuse of antibiotics in humans, this use of 'sub-therapeutic' levels of antibiotics in food animals may lead to serious health risks for people."[2] In 2002, the Alliance for the Prudent Use of Antibiotics (APUA) published a report titled "Facts About Antibiotics in Animals and Their Impact on Resistance," known as the FAAIR report.[3] The aim of the FAAIR project was to bring scientific evidence to the policy debate on antimicrobial use in agriculture and the risk it poses to human, animal, and ecological health. To meet this objective, the APUA convened a scientific advisory panel of experts from a variety of fields in research and medicine. Panel members analyzed relevant data from the scientific literature and developed consensus conclusions and policy recommendations. Many of the recommendations included in the FAAIR report have been largely ignored in the United States.

The use of antibiotics in feed is allowed in most developing countries, although the extent, level, and quality of the products used are difficult to assess. Illegal use is also widespread. Perhaps this situation should be expected in countries that have a poor public health infrastructure, but the situation is very similar in the developed countries. The Union of Concerned Scientists (UCS) estimates that 25 million lb of antibiotics is used every year in U.S. livestock for nontherapeutic purposes.[4] The breakdown is about 4 million lb in cattle, almost 11 million lb in swine, and 10 million lb in poultry. This figure has been challenged by the Animal Health Institute and many other individuals and agencies. However, it has been five years since the UCS report, and we still have little or no information regarding the actual totals of antibiotics used in livestock production. Given that many people believe there is a clear link between nontherapeutic use in livestock and antibiotic resistance, the time has come for full disclosure by the industry. At

Selected Antibiotics Approved for Use on Animals in the United States

Antibiotic Classes (selected examples)	Species	Disease Treatment	Disease Prevention	Growth Promotion
Aminoglycosides (gentamycin, neomycin, streptomycin)	beef cattle, goats, poultry, sheep, swine	×	×	
Beta-Lactams				
• penicillins (amoxicillin, ampicillin)	beef cattle, dairy cows, fowl, poultry, sheep, swine	×	×	×
• cephalosporins, 3rd generation (ceftiofur)	beef cattle, dairy cows, poultry, sheep, swine	×	×	
Chloramphenicol Florfenicol	beef cattle	×		
Ionophores (monensin, salinomycin, semduramicin, lasalocid)	beef cattle, fowl, goats, poultry, rabbits, sheep		×	×
Lincosamides (lincomycin)	poultry, swine	×	×	
Macrolides (erythromycin, tilmicosin, tylosin)	beef cattle, poultry, swine	×	×	×
Polypeptides (bacitracin)	fowl, poultry, swine	×	×	×
Quinolones Fluoroquinolones (sarafloxacin, enrofloxacin)	beef cattle	×	×	
Streptogramins (virginiamycin)	beef cattle, poultry, swine	×	×	×
Sulfonamides (sulfadimethoxine, sulfamethazine, sulfisoxazole)	beef cattle, dairy cows, fowl, poultry, swine, catfish, trout, salmon	×		×

(continued on next page)

**Selected Antibiotics Approved for Use
on Animals in the United States** *(continued)*

Antibiotic Classes *(selected examples)*	Species	Disease Treatment	Disease Prevention	Growth Promotion
Tetracyclines (chlortetracycline, oxytetracycline, tetracycline)	beef cattle, dairy cows, fowl, honey bees, poultry, sheep, swine, catfish, trout, salmon, lobster	×	×	×
Other antibiotics				
• Bambermycin	beef cattle, poultry, swine		×	×
• Carbadox	swine		×	×
• Novobiocin	fowl, poultry	×	×	
• Spectinomycin	poultry, swine		×	

Notes: An × indicates that the antibiotic use is approved. Poultry includes broiler chickens, laying hens, and turkeys. Fowl includes ducks, pheasants, and quail.

Source: Adapted from table II.1 in U.S. General Accounting Office, *Food Safety: The Agricultural Use of Antibiotics and Its Implications for Human Health* (Washington, D.C.: General Accounting Office, April 1999).

the very least, with accurate information, veterinary medicine can defend itself.

Attempts to Reduce Antibiotic Usage in Animal Production

There are many bacteria for which agriculture plays no part in the development of resistance. For example, the spread of a penicillin-resistant clone of *Streptococcus pneumoniae* has been driven exclusively by the use of penicillin in human medicine. However, it is much easier to disseminate antibiotic-resistant bacteria by global food distribution and inadequate waste management procedures than by person-to-person spread—and once resistant strains have developed, they appear to spread easily.

The use of antibiotics as growth promoters was recently banned in the EU and New Zealand, although since these bans went into effect there has been an increase in the use of antibiotics for therapeutic purposes. In Denmark, nontherapeutic antibiotics were banned in 2002, with no apparent apparent impact on animal health. Organic (antibiotic-free) farming has sometimes been suggested as a viable alternative. However, a number of studies suggest that organic farming is unlikely to be the solution. Fossler and colleagues concluded there was no significant difference in the prevalence of *Salmonella* on the organic and conventional farms they examined. In a similar study of *Salmonella* prevalence in swine, Gebreyes and colleagues found that the prevalence of *Salmonella* was significantly higher in animals from antibiotic-free farms (15.2 percent) than in animals from conventional farms (4.2 percent).[5,6]

Monitoring Antibiotic Resistance

It is important to understand international patterns of antibiotic resistance, and several surveillance projects have been initiated for this purpose. At present, most of the data published in the international literature on antimicrobial resistance are derived from short-term surveys of specific organisms and agents in defined areas. The consequences of this nonsystematic, discontinuous approach include the inability to establish meaningful baseline trends, low sensitivity in detecting new threats, inadequate information to evaluate interventions, and lack of data on organisms, antimicrobial drugs, and patient populations not included in the surveys.[7] The Global Advisory on Antibiotic Resistance Data (GAARD) is a consolidated group formed by the APUA that includes pharmaceutical company representation along with participation by the U.S. Centers for Disease Control and Prevention and WHO.[8,9] The aim of systems such as GAARD is to collect information from surveillance systems, and also to collect antibiotic use data where possible. One of the systems that provide data to GAARD is the SENTRY Antimicrobial Surveillance program. Bristol-Myers Squibb established the SENTRY program in 1997 as a global program for the surveillance of resistance in bacterial and fungal populations. It is the only global program that is monitoring changes in antibiotic resistance among human pathogens. The program is able to provide a snapshot of worldwide rates of antimicrobial resistance.

It is believed that the global food chain is a major vehicle for the spread of antibiotic-resistant bacteria. It is assumed that food intended for people and feed intended for animals are accidentally contaminated with feces during processing. However, people and animals can also be exposed to antibiotic drug residues and antibiotic-resistant bacteria as the result of coming into contact with animal wastes in open dumps. This is a major problem in the developing world.

References

1. World Health Organization (1996), Fighting Disease, Fostering Development, http://www.who.int/whr/1996/en/index.html.

2. Modern Meat (2002), http://www.pbs.org/wgbh/pages/frontline/shows/meat/.

3. FAAIR Advisory Panel (2002), "The Need to Improve Antimicrobial Use in Agriculture: Ecological and Human Health Effects," *Clinical Infectious Disease* 34 (Suppl.): 3.

4. Union of Concerned Scientists (2001), Hogging It! Estimates of Antimicrobial Use in Livestock (January), http://www.ucsusa.org/food_and_environment/antibiotics_and_food/hogging-it-estimates-of-antimicrobial-abuse-in-livestock.html.

5. C. P. Fossler, S. J. Wells, J. B. Kaneene, P. L. Ruegg, L. D. Warnick, J. B. Bender, S. M. Godden, C. W. Halbert, A. M. Campbell, and A. M. Zwald (2004), "Prevalence of *Salmonella* spp. on Conventional and Organic Dairy Farms," *Journal of the American Veterinary Medical Association* 225: 567–73.

6. W. A. Gebreyes, S. Thakur, and W. E. Morrow (2006), "Comparison of Prevalence, Antimicrobial Resistance, and Occurrence of Multidrug-Resistant *Salmonella* in Antimicrobial-Free and Conventional Pig Production," *Journal of Food Protection* 69: 743–48.

7. J. M. Stelling, K. Travers, R. N. Jones, P. J. Turner, T. F. O'Brien, and S. B. Levy (2005), "Integrating *Escherichia coli* Antimicrobial Susceptibility Data from Multiple Surveillance Programs," *Emerging Infectious Diseases* 11: 873–82.

8. GAARD Project (2005), http://www.tufts.edu/med/apua/Miscellaneous/GaardDesc.pdf.

9. World Health Organization (2003), Shaping the Future, http://www.who.int/whr/2003/en/.

Part III
Emerging Threats

Chapter 10
The Changing Epidemiology of Avian Influenza

Ilaria Capua, D. J. Alexander,
Bruce A. Rideout, and Martin Vincent

Avian influenza is the latest of a number of zoonotic diseases to emerge or reemerge in the past two decades. The majority of these emerging diseases originate in wildlife. Although the factors contributing to the emergence of these diseases are complex, the concept of ecological compartmentalization of disease agents provides a framework for understanding these processes.

Infectious agents are typically confined to certain host species, based on the life history traits of the host. These host factors effectively create ecological compartments that serve as barriers to the transmission of the agent to a novel host. If these natural ecological barriers are breached, the risk of cross-species transmission of disease increases. Zoos learned this lesson the hard way many decades ago when animals were commonly exhibited by taxonomic grouping, with little regard to whether or not they would normally come into contact in the wild. This situation created many opportunities for cross-species transmission of disease. Investigation of spontaneous disease outbreaks in zoos led to the characterization of a number of new host-adapted herpesviruses, adenoviruses, and other agents that were crossing over into new host species. This discovery led to the realization that animals should be exhibited based on shared biogeographic and ecological traits rather than on phylogenetic relationships. In other words, species should not be brought into contact in zoos if they do not come into contact in the wild. New strategies for exhibiting animals in naturalistic environments based on shared biogeographic and ecological traits have helped maintain these natural ecological barriers to disease transmission. This in turn has led to a reduction in disease transmission in zoos, resulting in significant improvement in the overall health and well-being of the animals.

We are now seeing the breakdown of ecological barriers to disease transmission in natural environments all over the world. Rapidly accelerating habitat loss, habitat fragmentation, and encroachment on wildlife and wildlife habitat by humans and domestic animals is bringing many different species into unnaturally close contact. As a result, there are many new opportunities for cross-species transmission of disease. This process may have contributed to the recent emergence of Henipah viruses in Australasia and severe acute respiratory syndrome (SARS) in Asia, and is now contributing to the uncontrolled spread of highly pathogenic avian influenza (HPAI) viruses.

Aquatic birds, particularly waterfowl, are the natural hosts for all low-pathogenicity avian influenza viruses.[1] The virus tends to be genetically stable in the natural host and does not normally cause disease. Susceptible hosts include poultry and nonaquatic birds. Poultry and other susceptible species become infected directly when they come into contact with infected reservoir species, or indirectly by the movement of infective secretions from the reservoir hosts to the susceptible hosts. This latter mechanism usually involves infective feces contaminating personnel or fomites that come in contact with susceptible hosts or the contamination of drinking water. Some AI strains of low pathogenicity have the potential to mutate to HPAI once they have infected susceptible poultry species. Devastating outbreaks often follow such mutational events, but domestic poultry have typically been dead-end hosts. Transmission of an HPAI strain back to wild aquatic birds is exceedingly rare, and sustained transmission does not normally occur in natural environments.

The ecological compartmentalization of avian influenza virus strains may be subtler than generally appreciated. Evidence suggests that certain virus strains circulate preferentially in gulls and terns that nest in large colonies.[2] In these species, virus transmission is most efficient during the nesting period, because that is when the greatest concentration of susceptible juveniles occurs. Other virus strains circulate preferentially in waterfowl, where the greatest concentration of susceptible juveniles occurs later in the season, during the summer molt. In wading birds, most influenza virus transmission probably occurs even later, with the highest virus prevalence occurring during spring migration. These life history traits tend to segregate the major transmission cycles of particular virus strains to particular host species, reducing opportunities for transmission across taxonomic groups.

Unfortunately, all of these subtle transmission dynamics are lost in parts of Asia where little separation occurs between domestic and wild birds, and this failure to maintain adequate barriers between domestic and wild birds is likely responsible for the first major outbreak of the H5N1 avian influenza in wildlife, which occurred at Qinghai Lake in central China in April 2005. More than 6,000 wild birds are estimated to have died in this outbreak, with bar-headed geese (*Anser indicus*) accounting for most of the mortality.[3,4,5] The westward spread of the virus following this outbreak was initially attributed to the movement of migratory birds, in part because the virus strain being spread was similar to the Qinghai Lake strain. However, this analysis failed to consider that migration generally occurs along routes that run north-south, not east-west. It also failed to consider the free exchange of viruses occurring between domestic and wild birds, and other avenues of movement that could create large geographic gaps between outbreaks. For example, circumstantial evidence now suggests that movement of domestic poultry and waterfowl on the Trans-Siberia Railway was an important contributor to the initial westward spread.[6]

This chapter describes our current understanding of how the H5N1 avian influenza virus emerged and was disseminated.

Classification and Mechanisms of Virulence

Influenza viruses have segmented, negative sense, single-strand RNA genomes and are placed in Family Orthomyxoviridae. At present, the Orthomyxoviridae family consists of five genera, but only viruses of the influenza virus A genus are known to infect birds. Influenza A viruses are further divided into subtypes based on the antigenic relationships in the surface glycoproteins, hemagglutinin (HA) and neuraminidase (NA). At present, sixteen HA subtypes (H1–H16) and nine NA subtypes (N1–N9) have been recognized. Each virus has one HA and one NA antigen, apparently in any combination. All influenza A subtypes in the majority of possible combinations have been isolated from avian species. To date, only viruses of H5 and H7 subtype have been shown to cause HPAI in susceptible species, but not all H5 and H7 viruses are virulent. For all influenza A viruses the HA glycoprotein is produced as a precursor, HA0, which requires posttranslational cleavage by host proteases before it is functional and virus particles are infectious.[7] The HA0 precursor proteins of avian influenza viruses of low virulence for poultry (LPAI viruses) have a single arginine at the cleavage site and another basic amino acid at position −3 or −4 from the cleavage site. These viruses are limited to cleavage by extracellular host proteases such as trypsin-like enzymes and are thus restricted to replication at sites in the host where such enzymes are found, that is, the respiratory and intestinal tracts. HPAI viruses possess multiple basic amino acids (arginine and lysine) at their HA0 cleavage sites as a result of either apparent insertion or apparent substitution,[8–10] and appear to be cleavable by an intracellular ubiquitous protease(s), probably one or more proprotein-processing subtilisin-related endoproteases, of which furin is the leading candidate.[11] HPAI viruses are able to replicate throughout the bird, damaging vital organs and tissues, which results in disease and death.

To date, only viruses of the H5 and H7 subtypes have been shown to cause HPAI. It appears that HPAI viruses arise by mutation after LPAI viruses have been introduced into poultry. Several mechanisms appear to be responsible for this mutation. Most HPAI viruses appear to have arisen as result of spontaneous duplication of purine triplets, which results in the insertion of basic amino acids at the HA0 cleavage site, and this apparently occurs due to a transcription fault by the polymerase complex.[12] However, as pointed out by Perdue and colleagues,[12] this is clearly not the only mechanism by which HPAI viruses arise, as some appear to result from nucleotide substitution rather than insertion, while others have insertions without repeating nucleotides. The Chile 2002[13] and the Canada 2004[14] H7N3 HPAI viruses show distinct and unusual cleavage site amino acid sequences. These viruses appear to have arisen as a result of recombination with other genes (nucleoprotein gene and matrix gene, respectively), resulting in an insertion at the cleavage site of 11 amino acids for the Chile virus and 7 amino acids for the Canadian virus.

The factors that bring about mutation from LPAI to HPAI are not known. In some instances, mutation seems to have taken place rapidly (at the primary site) after introduction from wild birds, in others the LPAI virus has circulated in poultry for months before mutating. Therefore, it is impossible to predict if and when this mutation will occur. However, it can be reasonably assumed that the wider the circulation of LPAI in poultry, the greater the chance that mutation to HPAI will occur. HPAI viruses are not necessarily virulent for all species of birds, and the clinical severity seen in any host appears to vary with both bird species and virus strain.[15,16] In particular, ducks rarely show clinical signs as a result of HPAI infections, although there are reports that some of the Asian H5N1 viruses have caused disease,[17] and the HPAI viruses A/duck/Italy/

2000 (H7N1) and A/chicken/Germany/34 (H7N1) have been reported to cause disease and death in naturally and experimentally infected waterfowl.[16]

Host Range

Influenza viruses have been shown to infect a great variety of birds,[18–22] including free-living birds, captive caged birds, domestic ducks, chickens, turkeys, and other domestic poultry. It was not until the mid-1970s that any systematic investigations of influenza in feral birds were undertaken. These investigations revealed enormous pools of influenza viruses to be present in the wild bird population,[2,22–24] especially in waterfowl, Family Anatidae, Order Anseriformes. In the surveys listed by Stallknecht and Shane,[24] a total of 21,318 samples from all species resulted in the isolation of 2,317 (10.9 percent) viruses. However, 14,303 of these samples were from birds of the Order Anseriformes, which yielded 2,173 (15.2 percent) isolates. The next highest isolation rates were 2.9 percent and 2.2 percent from the Passeriformes and Charadriiformes, respectively; but these compare with an overall isolation rate of 2.1 percent from all birds other than ducks and geese. However, studies by Sharp and colleagues[25] suggest that waterfowl do not act as a reservoir for all avian influenza viruses. It seems likely that part of the influenza gene pool is maintained in shorebirds and gulls, from which the predominant number of isolated influenza viruses are of a different subtype from those isolated from ducks.[26] Until the spread of Asian HPAI (H5N1), HPAI viruses had been isolated rarely from free-living birds and, apart from A/tern/S.Africa/61,[27] when they had been isolated it was usually in the vicinity of outbreaks of HPAI in poultry or geographically and chronologically close to known outbreaks in poultry. The different epidemiology of the Asian HPAI (H5N1) virus has led to several groups reexamining our understanding of avian influenza virus transmission. In particular, the change in the primary route of transmission from fecal-oral to the respiratory route in land birds, especially minor poultry species such as quail and pheasants, has been considered significant in the epidemiology of that virus, especially in its spread to mammals.[28–30]

The Emergence of the HPAI (H5N1) Virus

The emergence of the HPAI (H5N1) virus in Southeast Asia and its spread across Asia and into Europe and Africa is unprecedented in the virological era. The apparent progenitor virus for the subsequent outbreaks of HPAI of H5N1 subtype was obtained from an infection of commercial geese in Guandong province, People's Republic of China, in 1996.[31] In some reports it has been considered that the virus continued to circulate in southern China primarily in domestic ducks and showing some genetic variation.[32] This apparent low-level but probably endemic situation changed dramatically in December 2003 to February 2004, when suddenly eight countries in East and Southeast Asia reported outbreaks of HPAI due to H5N1 virus.[32] Although there seemed to be some success in controlling the outbreaks in some countries, it appeared to reemerge in a second wave from July 2004 on. Malaysia reported an outbreak in poultry in August 2004 and became the ninth country in the region to be affected.[33] The virus appeared to affect all sectors of the poultry populations in most of these countries, but its presence in free-range commercial ducks, village poultry, live bird markets, and fighting cocks seemed especially significant in the spread of the virus.[31,32,34] If HPAI virus becomes widespread in poultry, especially in domestic ducks that are reared on free range, spillover into wild bird populations is inevitable. In the past, such infections have been restricted to wild birds found dead in the vicinity of infected poultry, but there has always been concern that infections of wild birds in which HPAI virus caused minimal or no clinical signs (that is, ducks) could result in spread of the virus over large areas and long distances. Outbreaks affecting many wild bird species at two waterfowl parks in Hong Kong were recorded in 2002[35] and further, possibly more significant, outbreaks in wild migratory birds were reported in China and Mongolia in 2005. In particular, it was suggested that the presence of virus in migratory birds at Lake Qinghai in Western China could be the means by which the H5N1 virus could spread west and south.[36,37] But, as mentioned earlier, other movements, especially of poultry, may have been equally likely. There is no certain evidence that wild birds were responsible for the introduction into Russia, but HPAI (H5N1) virus, genetically closely related to isolates obtained at Lake Qinghai, reached poultry there in the summer of 2005. Whether spread from there to other West Asian and some East European countries occurred or whether the virus was introduced independently is not clear. Similarly, it is unclear whether spread was associated with movements of poultry or wild birds, since probably both were involved, but during 2005 and into the beginning of 2006, genetically closely related H5N1 viruses appeared in a number of countries in the region. Reports of HPAI H5N1 virus infections continued in Europe and in Africa during the first six months of 2006, and by the end of 2006, fifty-six countries in Asia, Europe, and Africa had reported HPAI caused by H5N1 virus to the World Organisation for Animal Health (OIE) since the end of 2003.[33]

Farming Systems in Developing Countries That Influence the Emergence of Avian Influenza

The emergence of HPAI, H5N1 strain in Asia and its subsequent spread to other continents is the result of years of fast and unregulated development of animal production systems to meet the increased demand in animal protein.[37] Highly concentrated domestic poultry production in densely populated regions, a rapid evolution of animal and farming production systems associated with centuries-old cultural practices that place humans and poultry in close mutual proximity, and the constant evolving nature of the virus have provided the ideal conditions for the emergence of new pathogenic strains of avian influenza virus.

In most countries in Southeast Asia, poultry production increased by 40 percent over the last decade. In Vietnam, for example, poultry production increased between 1990 and 2003 at an average annual rate of about 6 percent. Even so, increased production had trouble meeting demand until the onset of avian influenza. While per capita consumption of poultry meat is still very low in Vietnam (an estimated 3.9 kg per person in 2001), consumption doubled between 1990 and 2000, and high demand for poultry products among the rich (compared with demand for other livestock products) suggests strong future growth potential. The relatively low cost of raising poultry compared to raising cattle or pigs makes it the most popular livestock enterprise in rural households in Vietnam, where it is an important source of cash income, particularly for women. It is estimated that more than 70 percent of 12 million farming households keep poultry. Poultry is the most important livestock-based income source for the poorest quintile, with the sale of poultry products providing about 7 percent of cash income for these households. Poultry provides a form of savings that can be immediately available, and it is a relatively inexpensive protein source.[38] When farmers depend on their fowl for a subsistence living, they are naturally reluctant to destroy their flocks or to inform the authorities about sick birds, preferring to attempt to sell them or eat them.[39]

In Asia, production sectors can be divided according to the levels of biosecurity and trade. Sector 1 comprises industrial integrated systems with high level biosecurity and birds or products marketed commercially (for example, farms that are part of an integrated broiler production enterprise with clearly defined and implemented standard operating procedures for biosecurity). Sector 2 comprises commercial poultry production systems with moderate to high biosecurity and birds or products usually marketed commercially (for example, farms with birds kept indoors continuously, strictly preventing contact with other poultry or wildlife). Sector 3 consists of commercial poultry production systems with low to minimal biosecurity and birds or products entering live bird markets (examples of this category are a caged layer farm with birds in open sheds, a farm with poultry spending time outside the shed, or a farm producing chickens and waterfowl), and Sector 4 is made up of village or backyard production with minimal biosecurity and birds or products consumed locally. Small commercial farms and flocks of smallholders or villagers (sectors 3 and 4) appear to be more exposed to infection than larger commercial farms.[40] Numerically, more outbreaks occur in these smaller holdings even though, for a number of the infected countries, more poultry are raised in large farms. In Thailand, for example, a study of confirmed cases of HPAI (H5N1) infection from July to September 2004 demonstrated that some 64 percent of infected premises or holdings contained 1,000 or less poultry.[41] Within affected countries, disease appears to have spared many areas of high poultry population density, possibly reflecting the improved biosecurity and management practices of large industrial farms located in these areas. In many countries in Southeast Asia, although there are many industrial-level poultry operations, there are also many "backyard" flocks in which surveillance and biosecurity are minimal and farmers have little knowledge of the potential linkages of their activities to human infections with avian influenza.

It is also possible (though no firm evidence exists) that avian influenza may be spread by using chicken dung as food on fish farms, a common practice in Asia. Fertilizing fish ponds with poultry feces drastically improves fish growth and may set up major new reservoirs of avian influenza infection if the chickens or ducks providing the manure are infected themselves. Known as integrated livestock-fish farming, the technique involves transferring the wastes from raising pigs, ducks, or chickens directly to fish farms. At the right dosage, the nutrients in the manure give an enormous boost to the growth of plankton in the ponds, which are the main food of fish such as carp and tilapia. Furthermore, the management links between different ponds (such as the introduction of newly hatched fish) could also be a means of transmission of avian influenza virus. The long-distance transportation of poultry products for incorporation into fish feed, or already incorporated into exported fish feed, could provide additional opportunities for long-distance spread of the virus.[42]

Trade and Market Practices That May Affect the Emergence of Avian Influenza

Avian influenza viruses are known to spread readily as a result of the movement of infected poultry or contaminated equipment and clothing. These are considered important routes of spread for HPAI (H5N1) viruses in Asia, especially given the presence of these viruses in live bird markets and domestic waterfowl. In some countries, virus dissemination is facilitated by marketing and husbandry practices that result in mixing of different species of poultry in live bird markets and in some farms and villages. Transboundary trade in poultry and poultry products, both legal and illegal, is likely to have contributed to the spread of HPAI (H5N1) viruses. Long land borders exist between many of the infected countries in Southeast Asia, and smuggling of poultry and poultry products across many of these is acknowledged. Movement of live poultry (including fighting cocks) across borders is considered to be the most likely source of infection in some places. Much of the trade in live poultry involves day-old chicks. These birds are generally considered to be a relatively low risk because vertical transmission of HPAI (H5N1) viruses does not occur, and any residual virus on the surface of eggs would not normally survive the incubation process. Infected eggs would not hatch. The main risk associated with trade in day-old chicks arises from fomite transfer of infection via the re-use of transport crates, via vehicles, which could be contaminated outside of the hatchery, or by means of personnel involved in distribution.

As an example, HPAI (H5N1) is likely to have been introduced into Nigeria through the importation of day-old chicks. Trading patterns within countries also influence the spread of HPAI (H5N1) viruses. These differ considerably across the region, and work is ongoing to understand how this trade contributes to the spread of virus. As an example, trade in poultry in a country like Lao PDR is generally localized, with limited movement across the country. By contrast, extensive movements of poultry occur in China. Ducks raised in inland provinces in China are known to be sold in live birds markets in coastal provinces. Live poultry markets are recognized as important reservoirs of HPAI (H5N1) viruses if these are managed using a continuous flow system, and especially if poultry are allowed to remain for longer than 24 hours in the markets. They are likely to play an important role in the maintenance and more particularly in the dissemination of HPAI in countries where this practice is widespread. However, additional studies need to be undertaken to fully assess the impact of local trading patterns on the distribution of H5N1 HPAI viruses. Such studies have already started in Vietnam and Indonesia, where value market studies are looking at risk factors and corrective measures along the market chains.

Role of Waterfowl and Wetlands in the Emergence of Avian Influenza

Domestic waterfowl are believed to have played a key role in the genesis of the 2003–2004 epidemics. Much of this can be ascribed to the ability of asymptomatic ducks to carry early strains of HPAI (H5N1) viruses. As noted above, carriage of these viruses by healthy ducks is not a unique feature of the HPAI (H5N1) viruses circulating in Asia. In Vietnam and Thailand, they are believed to play a key role in the maintenance of infection, especially free-grazing ducks associated with rice production cycles.[42,43]

The importance of waterfowl in the emergence of HPAI (H5N1) virus has focused attention on the role of wetlands. Wetland losses over the past two centuries have been severe. In the United States, it is estimated that a 53 percent decline in wetlands occurred between 1780 and 1980.[44] In Natal Province in South Africa, the Tugela Basin has seen the loss of more than 90 percent of its wetlands, while in the Mfolozi catchment approximately 58 percent of the wetlands have been destroyed.[39] The situation in densely populated regions of Southeast Asia differs from much of the rest of the world in that extensive wetland loss has occurred over a very long period of time, going back six millennia, as lowland rice cultivation was established about 6,500 years ago.[45] Indeed, over the millennia, vast areas of wetland in southern and eastern Asia were converted into rice fields or drained for other forms of agriculture and human settlement. It is also assumed that almost all of the 40 million hectares of rice cultivation in the central plains of India were developed at the expense of natural wetlands, as were the 1.9 million hectares of rice cultivation in the central plains of Thailand. In all of these regions, very little natural wetland vegetation has survived into the present.[45,46] Thus cultural practices and environmental change have resulted in more commingling of domestic poultry and wild birds at watering and feeding grounds. In Southeast Asia, the large-scale and ongoing elimination of natural wetlands cannot help but encourage further mixing of wild migrating birds with domestic fowl. This may well be of particular concern in the lowlands of China, where the loss of natural wetlands over the centuries has created vast agricultural areas providing food and water for both domestic and wild birds. Such situations provide ideal conditions for HPAI virus to move from wild birds into domestic flocks.

Cultural Practices and Religious Festivals and Ceremonies in the Emergence of Avian Influenza

The Tet Nguyen Dan or Tet festival, which means the Lunar New Year, is a festival that is celebrated in Vietnam and starts on the first day of the first lunar month. Tet marks the end of the lunar calendar and the beginning of spring. This is the occasion of major family gathering and celebrations and traditionally involves the consumption of chicken as part of ceremonial offerings. Poultry production and demand increase markedly before this period as well as for trade during the festival. The Tet festival usually takes place in February and leads to increased animal and human movements. In Vietnam, the peak of HPAI outbreaks was observed during two consecutive years before and during the Tet festival period, which certainly played a major role in the spread of the disease.

Today, some cultural practices may lend themselves extremely well to the emergence of new pathogens. The open question is, will and can there be rapid adaptation in various cultures, both in the East and in the West, to recognize the considerable risks to human health from present farming and animal husbandry practices? It is not just a matter of ancient practices in the East coupled with growing populations but also consumption demand in the West, fueling expanding trade; both need to change.[39]

The Role of Migratory Birds in Disseminating Avian Influenza Virus

It is thought that migratory birds may not have played a significant role in the original westward spread of the virus from Southeast Asia; however, there is epidemiological evidence of subsequent spread by wild birds from the West Siberian Lowlands southward along the Black Sea–Mediterranean flyway.[40,41] The best circumstantial evidence for virus spread by wild birds is the occurrence of outbreaks in wild birds in countries not experiencing poultry outbreaks (such as Italy in late 2005 and early 2006). Although migratory birds are now moving the virus, it is widely recognized that the movement of poultry, poultry products, and domestic waterfowl is primarily responsible for the ongoing spread in poultry.[47] The primary concern with the presence of HPAI (H5N1) virus in wild bird populations is the potential to increase the number of viral reservoirs to an extent that will make eradication impossible. In addition, frequent cross-species transmission increases the risk of viral recombination events, which contributes to ongoing strain evolution and the potential for a new pandemic strain to arise.

Conclusion

The epidemiology of AI has changed in the last 10 years, not only because of the failure to control and eradicate infections in poultry due to HPAI (H5N1) viruses, but also because the continued global development and industrialization of the poultry industries have meant that avian influenza infections, especially HPAI outbreaks, have had a far greater impact in terms of spread and loss of birds than in earlier years. The spread of HPAI virus to wild birds on the scale reached by the Asian HPAI (H5N1) virus is unprecedented. Whether the virus is likely to become or remain endemic in some species of wild birds or will gradually die out if there is no further spread from infected poultry is not clear. This change in the ecology and epidemiology of avian influenza infections requires the urgent generation of new knowledge on issues related to epidemiology, pathogenesis, and control. The Asian HPAI (H5N1) viruses have spread to three continents with completely different agricultural, ecological, social, and economic backgrounds. This in turn is likely to result in the establishment of different mechanisms by which the virus may be perpetuated in a given area. The generation of such cycles will be influenced by the diversity and availability of hosts in that area. As the virus encounters new hosts, within and outside the Class *Aves*, it may well acquire mutations that may reflect replication advantages in one or more species but affect the pathogenicity and transmissibility in those and other species.

What then can be done to stop the uncontrolled spread of H5N1 avian influenza? Most of the response effort has focused on early detection and eradication programs for poultry, as well as prevention through vaccination.[47] Little attention has been given to the importance of reestablishing the normal ecological barriers to cross species transmission. More effort should be directed to establishment of transmission barriers between wild and domestic waterfowl. There is mounting evidence that asymptomatic infection of domestic waterfowl was a major factor in the original spread of the virus throughout Asia.[34,41,48] Ongoing transmission between domestic and wild waterfowl is now contributing to the uncontrolled spread in wildlife, including spillover to novel hosts such as nonaquatic birds, wild carnivores, and domestic pets. Developing countries need simple but effective means of establishing better buffers between agricultural species and wildlife. In addition, suitable wetland habitat needs to be preserved for wildlife as protected breeding grounds and migratory stopover points. Finally, better regional biosecurity is needed to prevent the movement of disease agents and vectors across borders, whether it is the movement of domestic poultry and waterfowl products or smuggled wildlife. Greater attention must be paid to the ways in which human encroachment on wildlife is influencing the emergence of new zoonoses, such as H5N1 avian influenza. This will be one of the great challenges to veterinary medicine and public health in the twenty-first century.

References

1. D. J. Alexander (2000), "A Review of Avian Influenza in Different Bird Species," *Veterinary Microbiology* 74: 3–13.
2. B. Olsen, V. J. Munster, A. Wallensten, J. Waldenstrom, A. D. Osterhaus, and R. A. Fouchier (2006), "Global Patterns of Influenza A Virus in Wild Birds," *Science* 312, no. 5772: 384–88.
3. H. Chen, G. J. D. Smith, S. Y. Zhang, K. Qin, J. Wang, K. S. Li, R. G. Webster, J. S. M. Peiris, and Y. Guan (2005), "H5N1 Virus Outbreak in Migratory Waterfowl," *Nature* 436: 191–92.
4. J. Y. Zhou, H. G. Shen, H. X. Chen, G. Z. Tong, M. Liao, H. C. Yang, and J. X. Liu (2006), "Characterization of a Highly Pathogenic H5N1 Influenza Virus Derived from Bar-Headed Geese in China," *Journal of General Virology* 87: 1823–33.
5. D. Butler (2006), "Blogger Reveals China's Migratory Goose Farms near Site of Flu Outbreak," *Nature* 441: 263.
6. J. McConnell (2006), "The *Lancet* Forum on Preparing for Pandemic Influenza," *Lancet Infectious Diseases* 6, no. 7: 390–92.
7. R. Rott (1992), "The Pathogenic Determinant of Influenza Virus," *Veterinary Microbiology* 33: 303–10.
8. M. Vey, M. Orlich, S. Adler, H. D. Klenk, R. Rott, and W. Garten (1992), "Haemagglutinin Activation of Pathogenic Avian Influenza Viruses of Serotype H7 Requires the Recognition Motif R-X-R/K-R," *Virology* 188: 408–13.
9. G. W. Wood, J. W. McCauley, J. B. Bashiruddin, and D. J. Alexander (1993), "Deduced Amino Acid Sequences at the Haemagglutinin Cleavage Site of Avian Influenza A Viruses of H5 and H7 Subtypes," *Archives of Virology* 130: 209–17.
10. D. A. Senne, B. Panigrahy, Y. Kawaoka, J. E. Pearson, J. Suss, M. Lipkind, H. Kida, and R. G. Webster (1996), "Survey of the Hemagglutinin (HA) Cleavage Site Sequence of H5 and H7 Avian Influenza Viruses: Amino Acid Sequence at the HA Cleavage Site as a Marker of Pathogenicity Potential," *Avian Diseases* 40: 425–37.
11. A. Stieneke-Grober, M. Vey, H. Angliker, E. Shaw, G. Thomas, C. Roberts, H. D. Klenk, and W. Garten (1992), "Influenza Virus Hemagglutinin with Multibasic Cleavage Site is Activated by Furin, a Subtilisin Endoprotease," *EMBO Journal* 11: 2407–14.

12. M. Perdue, J. Crawford, M. Garcia, J. Latimer, and D. E. Swayne (1998), "Occurrence and Possible Mechanisms of Cleavage Site Insertions in the Avian Influenza Hemagglutinin Gene," in *Proceedings of the 4th International Symposium on Avian Influenza* (Athens, Ga.: U.S. Animal Health Association), 182–93.

13. D. L. Suarez, D. A. Senne, J. Banks, I. H. Brown, S. C. Essen, C. W. Lee, R. J. Manvell, C. Mathieu-Benson, V. Mareno, J. Pedersen, B. Panigrahy, H. Rojas, E. Spackman, and D. J. Alexander (2004), "Recombination Resulting in Virulence Shift in Avian Influenza Outbreak, Chile," *Emerging Infectious Diseases* 10: 1–13.

14. J. Pasick, K. Handel, J. Robinson, J. Copps, D. Ridd, K. Hills, H. Kehler, C. Cottam-Birt, J. Neufeld, Y. Berhane, and S. Czub (2005), "Intersegmental Recombination Between the Haemagglutinin and Matrix Genes Was Responsible for the Emergence of a Highly Pathogenic H7N3 Avian Influenza Virus in British Columbia," *Journal of General Virology* 86: 727–31.

15. D. J. Alexander, W. H. Allan, D. Parsons, and G. Parsons (1978), "The Pathogenicity of Four Avian Influenza Viruses for Chickens, Turkeys and Ducks," *Research in Veterinary Science* 24: 242–47.

16. I. Capua and F. Mutinelli (2001), "Mortality in Muscovy Ducks (*Cairina moschata*) and Domestic Geese (*Anser* var. *domestica*) Associated with Natural Infection with a Highly Pathogenic Avian Influenza Virus of H7N1 Subtype," *Avian Pathology* 30(2): 179–83.

17. K. M. Sturm-Ramirez, D. J. Hulse-Post, E. A. Govorkova, J. Humberd, P. Seiler, P. Puthavathana, C. Buranathai, T. D. Nguyen, A. Chaisingh, H. T. Long, T. S. P. Naipospos, H. Chen, T. M. Ellis, Y. Guan, J. S. M. Peiris, and R. G. Webster (2005), "Are Ducks Contributing to the Endemicity of Highly Pathogenic H5N1 Influenza Virus in Asia?" *Journal of Virology* 79: 11269–79.

18. D. K. Lvov (1978), "Circulation of Influenza Viruses in Natural Biocenosis," in *Viruses and Environment*, ed. E. Kurstak and K. Maramovosch (New York: Academic Press), 351–80.

19. V. S. Hinshaw, R. G. Webster, and J. Rodriguez (1981), "Influenza A Viruses: Combinations of Haemagglutinin and Neuraminidase Subtypes Isolated from Animals and Other Sources," *Archives of Virology* 67: 191–206.

20. D. J. Alexander (2001), "Ecology of Avian Influenza in Domestic Birds," in *Proceedings of the International Symposium on Emergence and Control of Zoonotic Ortho- and Paramyxovirus Diseases*, ed. B. Dodet and M. Vicari (Veyrier-du-lac, France: Merieux Foundation), 25–34.

21. D. J. Alexander (2000), "A Review of Avian Influenza in Different Bird Species," in *Proceedings of the ESVV Symposium on Animal Influenza Viruses, Gent 1999, Veterinary Microbiology* 74: 3–13.

22. ESFA Scientific Panel on Animal Health and Animal Welfare (2005), "Animal Health and Welfare Aspects of Avian Influenza," Annex to *EFSA Journal* 266: 1–21.

23. D. E. Stallknecht (1998), "Ecology and Epidemiology of Avian Influenza Viruses in Wild Bird Populations," in *Proceedings of the Fourth International Symposium on Avian Influenza* (Athens, Ga.: U.S. Animal Health Association), 61–69.

24. D. E. Stallknecht and S. M. Shane (1988), "Host Range of Avian Influenza Virus in Free-Living Birds," *Veterinary Research Communications* 12: 125–41.

25. G. B. Sharp, Y. Kawaoka, S. M. Wright, B. Turner, V. S. Hinshaw, and R. G. Webster (1993), "Wild Ducks Are the Reservoir for Only a Limited Number of Influenza A Subtypes," *Epidemiology and Infection* 110: 161–76.

26. Y. Kawaoka, T. M. Chambers, W. L. Sladen, and R. G. Webster (1988), "Is the Gene Pool of Influenza Viruses in Shorebirds and Gulls Different from That in Wild Ducks?" *Virology* 163: 247–50.

27. W. B. Becker (1966), "The Isolation and Classification of Tern Virus: Influenza Virus A/Tern/South Africa/1961," *Journal of Hygiene* 64: 309–20.

28. D. R. Perez, R. J. Webby, and R. G. Webster (2003), "Land-Based Birds as Potential Disseminators of Avian/Mammalian Reassortant Influenza A Viruses," *Avian Diseases* 47: 1114–17.

29. N. V. Mararova, H. Ozaki, H. Kida, R. G. Webster, and D. R. Perez (2003), "Replication and Transmission of Influenza Viruses in Japanese Quail," *Virology* 310: 8–15.

30. J. Humbred, Y. Guan, and R. G. Webster (2006), "Comparison of the Replication of Influenza A Viruses in Chinese Ring-Necked Pheasants and Chukar Partridges," *Journal of Virology* 80: 2151–61.

31. X. Xu, K. Subbarao, N. J. Cox, and Y. Guo (1999), "Genetic Characterization of the Pathogenic Influenza A/Goose/Guandong/1/96 (H5N1) Virus: Similarity of Its Haemagglutinin Gene to Those of H5N1 Viruses from the 1997 Outbreaks in Hong Kong," *Virology* 261: 15–19.

32. L. D. Sims, J. Domench, C. Benigno, S. Kahn, A. Kamaya, J. Lubroth, V. Martin, and P. Roeder (2005), "Origin and Evolution of Highly Pathogenic H5N1 Avian Influenza in Asia," *Veterinary Record* 157: 159–64.

33. OIE (2006), Update on Avian Influenza in Animals (type H5), April 7, http://www.oie.int/downld/AVIAN%20INFLUENZA/A_AI-Asia.htm.

34. T. Songserm, R. Jam-on, N. Sae-Heng, N. Meemak, D. J. Hulse-Post, K. M. Sturm-Ramirez, and R. G. Webster (2006), "Domestic Ducks and H5N1 Influenza Epidemic, Thailand," *Emerging Infectious Diseases* 12: 1–12.

35. T. M. Ellis, R. B. Bousfield, L. A. Bissett, K. C. Dyrting, G. S. M. Luk, S. T. Tsim, K. Sturm-Ramirez, R. G. Webste, Y. Guan, and J. S. M. Peiris (2002), "Investigation of Outbreaks of Highly Pathogenic H5N1 Avian Influenza in Waterfowl and Wild Birds in Hong Kong in Late 2002," *Avian Patholology* 33: 492–505.

36. H. Chen, G. J. D. Smith, S. Y. Zhang, K. Qin, J. Wang, K. S. Li, R. G. Webster, J. S. M. Peiris, and Y. Guan (2005), "H5N1 Virus Outbreak in Migratory Waterfowl," *Nature* 436: 191–92.

37. V. Martin, L. Sims, J. Lubroth, D. Pfeiffer, J. Slingenbergh, and J. Domenech (2006), "Epidemiology and Ecology of Highly Pathogenic Avian Influenza with Particular Emphasis on South East Asia," *Developments in Biologicals* 124: 23–36.

38. Agrifood Consulting International (2006), *The Impact of Avian Influenza on Poultry Sector Restructuring and Its Socio-Economic Effects* (Bethesda, Md.: AGI).

39. D. J. Rapport (2006), "Avian Influenza and the Environment: An Ecohealth Perspective," presented at the Scientific Seminar on Avian Influenza, the Environment, and Migratory Birds, UNEP Headquarters, Gigiri, Nairobi, April 10–11.

40. M. Gilbert, X. Xiao, J. Domenech, J. Lubroth, V. Martin, and J. Slingenbergh (2006), HPAI Spread from the West Siberian Lowland to the Eastern Mediterranean and Beyond, FAO Report (February).

41. M. Gilbert, P. Chaitaweesub, T. Parakamawongsa, S. Premashthira, T. Tiensin, W. Kalpravidh, H. Wagner, and J. Slingenbergh (2006), "Free-Grazing Ducks and Highly Pathogenic Avian Influenza, Thailand," *Emerging Infectious Diseases* 2: 227–34.

42. C. J. Feare (2006), *Fish Farming and the Risk of Spread of Avian Influenza* (London: Birdlife International).

43. D. U. Pfeiffer (2005), *Geospatial Analysis of HPAI Outbreaks in Vietnam* (Rome: FAO).

44. T. E. Dahl (1990), *Wetlands Losses in the United States 1780s to 1980s* (Washington, D.C.: U.S. Department of the Interior, Fish and Wildlife Service).

45. M. Moser, C. Prentice, and S. Frazier (1996) (Wetlands International), "A Global Overview of Wetland Loss and Degradation," presented to technical session B of the 6th meeting of the conference of the contracting parties, Brisbane, Australia, March 1996, *Conference Proceedings*, vol. 10.

46. D. A. Scott (1993), "Wetland Inventories and the Assessment of Wetland Loss: A Global Overview," in *Waterfowl and Wetland Conservation in the 1990s: A Global Perspective: Proceedings of the IWRB Symposium, St. Petersburg, Florida, 12–19 November 1992*, ed. M. Moser, R. C. Prentice, and J. van Vessem, IWRB Special Publication 26 (Slimbridge, UK: International Waterfowl and Wetlands Research Bureau).

47. World Health Organization (2006), Influenza Research at the Human and Animal Interface, Working Group Report (Geneva: WHO, September).

48. K. S. Li, Y., Guan, J. Wang, G. J. D. Smith, K. M. Xu, L. Duan, A. P. Rahardjo, P. Puthavathana, C. Buranathai, T. D. Nguyen, A. T. S. Estoepangestie, A. Chaisingh, P. Auewarakul, H. T. Long, N. T. H. Hanh, R. J. Webby, L. L. M. Poon, H. Chen, K. F. Shortridge, K. Y. Yuen, R. G. Webster, and J. S. M. Peiris (2004), "Genesis of a Highly Pathogenic and Potentially Pandemic H5N1 Influenza Virus in Eastern Asia," *Nature* 430: 209–13.

Chapter 11
Wildlife Zoonoses
Emerging and Reemerging Zoonoses
from Wildlife Reservoirs

Bruno B. Chomel

Emerging infectious diseases are characterized by the identification of formerly unknown disease agents and the diseases they cause, or the global dispersion of known pathogens, as well as the observation of increasing resistance to antibiotics.[1] It is estimated that 75 percent of the emerging infectious diseases are zoonotic, mainly of viral origin, and likely to be vector-borne.[2] Infectious pathogens of wildlife have become increasingly important worldwide, as they have major impacts not only on human health and agricultural production but also on wildlife-based economies and wildlife conservation. Zoonotic pathogens that can infect both domestic animals and wildlife hosts are more likely to emerge.[3] As stated by Bengis and colleagues, "the emergence of these wildlife pathogens is associated with a range of causal factors, most of them linked to the sharp and exponential rise of global human activity. Among these causal factors are the burgeoning human population, the increased frequency and speed of local and international travel, the increase in human-assisted movement of animals and animal products, changing agricultural practices that favor the transfer of pathogens between wild and domestic animals, and a range of environmental changes that alter the distribution of wild hosts and vectors and thus facilitate the transmission of infectious agents."[4]

The Economic Importance of Wildlife and Wildlife Trade

Wildlife is a source of major economic income either in direct values, such as consumptive or productive use values, or indirect values, such as touristic and scientific values (wildlife safaris, bird watching), not to mention ethical and optional values, as defined by McNeely and colleagues.[5] The consumptive and nonconsumptive uses of wildlife are a major revenue source in the annual gross product of many developing countries, especially in Africa and Asia, accounting for millions to hundred of millions of U.S. dollars.[6] In the United States, it was estimated that total expenditure for wildlife-related activities was U.S. $101 billion in 1996, approximately 1.4 percent of the national economy.[6] In the United States, hunting activities generated more than 700,000 jobs and several billions of dollars in state and federal tax revenue.[6] The estimate for trade and local and regional consumption of wild animal meat in Central Africa alone is more than one billion kg per year.[7]

The exponential growth of the human population, from less than one billion humans at the beginning of the last century to 6.5 billion in 2006, has led to major ecological changes, with a drastic reduction in wildlife natural habitats associated with human population encroachment on these habitats.[8] Human activities also appear to create important climatic changes referred to as global warming, which is characterized by a dramatic reduction of the glaciers worldwide, a reduction of the polar ice caps, a warming trend in usually temperate climates with heavy rainfall, and the spread of vector-borne diseases, such as malaria, dengue, or Japanese encephalitis. Correlations between warmer, wetter conditions associated with El Niño events and outbreaks of malaria, dengue, Rift Valley fever, Hantaviruses, and plague have been demonstrated.[9] Among the many examples of the emergence or reemergence of zoonotic diseases related to human encroachment on wildlife habitat are the increasing number of human cases of rabies related to vampire bat rabies in the Amazon Basin,[10–15] the emergence of tick-borne zoonoses, such as Lyme disease and the ehrlichioses in North America[16] and Kyasanur Forest virus in India,[17] and also some parasitic diseases, such as that caused by *Baylisascaris procyonis*.[18] Deforestation and the development of human habitat, as well as mining activities, have been suggested as risk factors associated with the recent reemergence of vampire bat rabies in humans in the Amazon Basin.[10,12,14,15] In 2004, forty-six persons died of rabies caused by vampire bats, mainly in Brazil (twenty-two cases) and Colombia (fourteen cases); whereas only twenty human cases of rabies were transmitted by dogs in Latin America.[13]

The reduction of traditional agricultural land and its substitution by forested areas, where the main reservoirs and hosts of *Borrelia burgdorferi* live, in association with the settlement of people in peri-urban areas has led to a considerable increase in human cases of Lyme disease.[19,20] It is estimated that approximately 32.4 million deer, elk, antelope, and other wild ruminants, which are major amplifiers for adult *Ixodes scapularis* ticks, live in North America.[21] Similarly, although the number of human cases is limited but associated with severe neurological symptoms, infection by embryonated eggs of *B. procyonis* has been on the increase in areas where raccoon populations are on the increase, especially in coastal California.[22] The geographic distribution of raccoons is expanding and their numbers in urban and suburban areas are increasing.[23] Raccoon latrines are usually close to human settings and are recognized as an important potential source of human infection. In India, when first described in 1957, Kyasanur Forest disease was restricted to a much smaller area (300 square miles) than the actual 2,000 square miles of endemic zone.[17] It is a tick-borne disease present in a region of evergreen rain forest interspersed with deciduous patches and clearings for rice cultivation and human habitations. Most human cases occur during the dry season (January–May), when nymphal activity is maximal. Such a zoonosis is a good example of deforestation and agricultural development leading to human habitat expansion into natural foci of a viral infection. As cleared areas have been widely used for cattle grazing, it favored the proliferation of the tick *Haemaphysalis spinigera*, as cattle are a major host for adult ticks. Thus, a latent zoonosis was transformed into an epidemic.[17] Human activities may also be a source of wildlife infection that may lead to creating new reservoirs of human pathogens. The recent outbreak of tuberculosis caused by *Mycobacterium tuberculosis* in suricats and mongooses was one of the first documented spillovers of a human disease within a wildlife population.[24] Banded mongooses were observed feeding regularly at garbage pits and would therefore have been exposed to human excretions and any infectious material from tuberculosis-infected humans. In recent years, outbreaks of tuberculosis caused by *M. tuberculosis* have been reported in captive elephants in the United States and Sweden, and at several locations human exposures to infection were documented.[25,26] The reemergence of zoonotic diseases that had been eradicated from their domestic animal reservoirs is also of major concern. Wildlife may become a new reservoir of infection and recontaminate domestic animal.[4] Such examples are well illustrated by the reemergence of bovine tuberculosis in the UK, associated with the presence of *M. bovis* infection in badgers (*Meles meles*)[27] and in Michigan associated with a large outbreak within the local deer population,[28] or by the reemergence of brucellosis in swine in Europe as a result of spillover from the wild boar brucellosis (*Brucella suis biovar* 2) reservoir, particularly in outdoor-reared pigs.[29,30]

Changes in Agricultural Practices and the Emergence of Wildlife Zoonoses

The outbreak of Nipah virus in Malaysia in 1998–1999, which caused 265 human cases of viral encephalitis with a 38 percent mortality, was the result of several major ecological and environmental changes associated with deforestation and the expansion of pig farming in rather primitive settings, in association with production of fruit-bearing trees.[31] Such a combination led to the infection of pigs, which developed respiratory and neurological symptoms following exposure to infected fruit bats, likely to shed the virus in their urine and feces. Then the sick pigs became a source of human infection.[31] Farming of new animal species has led to the emergence or reemergence of zoonoses such as bovine tuberculosis in captive deer populations[32] or Eastern equine encephalitis in emus.[33] Deer at low population densities on natural range are generally not affected by disease to any significant extent. However, they are susceptible to many diseases, and hence disease becomes an important factor in the intensive management of deer. *Yersinia* pseudotuberculosis has been recognized as a major cause of death in farmed deer.[34] Outbreaks were manifested by gastroenteritis and the sudden death of deer of all ages, but mainly young deer. Tuberculosis has also been recorded among various deer species; it can become widespread among farmed deer if testing and slaughter of reactors is not conducted.[32]

Trade in wildlife provides disease transmission mechanisms at levels that not only cause human disease outbreaks but also threaten livestock, international trade, rural livelihoods, native wildlife populations, and the health of ecosystems.[7,8] Some estimates indicate that about 40,000 live primates, 4 million live birds, 640,000 live reptiles, and 350 million live tropical fishes are traded globally each year.[7] It is estimated that the international wildlife trade is a U.S. $6 billion industry.[35] Translocation of wild animals has been associated with the spread of several zoonoses. Rabies was introduced in the mid-Atlantic states in the 1970s by repopulating hunting pens with raccoons trapped in rabies-endemic zones of the southern United States.[19] In Finland, an outbreak of rabies occurred in raccoon dogs in 1988, as this wildlife species spread in new habitats from the accidental release of animals raised for the fur trade.[19] This species appears to constitute a new reservoir of rabies in Eastern Europe, besides the red fox reservoir. Similarly, translocation of hares from Hungary, Slovakia, and the Czech Republic for sporting purposes has led to several outbreaks of tularemia and the introduction of *Brucella suis biovar* 2 in Western Europe[36] and its encroachment on the wild boar population.[29] For the period 1993–2003, *B. suis biovar* 2 infections were reported on more than forty outdoor rearing pig farms in France.[29] Similarly, *Echinococcus multi-*

locularis was detected in red foxes (*Vulpes vulpes*) illegally imported into South Carolina (United States) for release in fox-chasing enclosures[37] and was recently detected in Norway, probably following its introduction by migrating arctic foxes and its establishment through accidental translocation of the intermediate host, the sibling vole.[19] Many years ago, brush-tailed possums (*Trichosurus vulpecula*) from Tasmania were introduced into New Zealand to establish a new species of fur-bearer. The translocated population proliferated and is now estimated to be over 70 million, of which 3 to 30 percent are possibly infected by *M. bovis*, a permanent threat to the cattle and deer farming industries.[36] Wild populations of introduced species can also become common disease reservoirs, a role played by Indian mongooses (*Herpestes javanicus*) in rabies transmission on some Caribbean islands.[38] Illegal trade can also be a source of human infection. In March 1994, health authorities in Antwerp, Belgium, were informed that a member of a team of fifteen customs officers had developed psittacosis.[39] The customs officer concerned had been admitted to hospital with pneumonia 10 days after exposure to parakeets that had been imported illegally by an Indian sailor. The risk of contracting psittacosis was 2.8 times higher in officers exposed for more than 2 hours to parakeets than for those briefly exposed. Similarly, isolation and characterization of the highly pathogenic avian influenza A virus, H5N1 strain, was reported from Crested Hawk-Eagles smuggled into Europe by air travel.[40] Luckily, screening performed in human and avian contacts indicated no dissemination occurred.

The Bushmeat Market, Live Animal Markets, and Exotic Foods

Another risk factor related to the emergence of zoonotic diseases from wildlife has been the considerable increase in bushmeat consumption in many parts of the world, especially in Central Africa, where an estimated 1 to 3.4 million tons are consumed annually, and in the Amazon Basin, where an estimated 67 to 164 million kg of bushmeat is consumed annually.[8,41] The simian foamy virus has been identified as a retroviral zoonosis in people who have direct contact with fresh nonhuman primate bushmeat, which suggests that such zoonoses are more frequent, widespread, and contemporary than previously appreciated. Similarly, new retroviruses, human T-lymphotropic virus (HTLV) type 3 and type 4, were found in people who hunt, butcher, or keep monkeys or apes as pets in southern Cameroon.[41] The increased amount of hunting in Africa that has resulted from a combination of urban demand for bushmeat (a multi-billion-dollar business) and greater access to primate habitats provided by logging roads, has increased the frequency of human exposure to primate retroviruses and other disease-causing agents.[42] Similarly, most of the recent outbreaks of Ebola virus in western Africa have been associated with consumption of bushmeat (mainly dead chimpanzees).[43]

Traditional and local food markets in many parts of the world can be associated with emergence of new zoonotic diseases. Live animal markets, also known as "wet markets," have always been the principal mode of commercialization of poultry and many other animals, including small carnivores, amphibians, and reptiles. The avian influenza epidemic that has plagued Southeast Asia since 2003 and is spreading in other parts of the world is directly related to infected birds sold live in traditional markets and facilitates the spread of this avian H5N1 virus by wild birds.[44] Similarly, the newly discovered severe acute respiratory syndrome (SARS)-associated coronavirus has been linked to the live trade of wild carnivores, especially civets, in China.[45] However, civet may only be an amplifier of the SARS coronavirus endemic in wild Chinese horseshoe bats.[46] If trichinellosis has long been associated with the consumption of undercooked meat from wild animals, such as bears,[47] consumption of uncooked venison (deer and wild boar) has been more recently associated with the emergence of severe cases of hepatitis E in hunters in Japan.[48] The new taste in developed nations for "trendy" exotic food as also been linked with different zoonotic food-borne pathogens or parasites. As stated by MacPherson, "The increasing proclivity for eating meat, fish, crabs, shrimp, molluscs raw, undercooked, smoked, pickled or dried facilitates a number of protozoan (*Toxoplasma*), trematode (*Fasciola* sp., *Paragonimus* spp., *Clonorchis* sp., *Opisthorchis* spp., *Heterophyes* sp., *Metagonimus* sp., *Echinostoma* spp., *Nanophyetus* sp.), cestode (*Taenia* spp, *Diphyllobothrum* sp.), and nematode (*Trichinella* spp., *Capillaria* spp., *Gnathostoma* spp., *Anisakis* sp., *Parastrongylus* spp.) caused zoonoses."[49]

Ecotourism

Adventure travel is now the largest growing segment of the leisure travel industry, with a growth rate of 10 percent per year since 1985 (Adventure Travel Society, pers. comm.). This type of travel has led to an increasing risk for contact with pathogens uncommon in industrialized countries, especially for participants in adventure sports and extreme travel. An outbreak of leptospirosis was diagnosed and all ill persons had participated in the Eco-Challenge-Sabah 2000 multisport 10-day endurance race, held in Malaysian Borneo, where 304 athletes from twenty-seven countries competed. Segments of the event included jungle trekking, prolonged swimming and kayaking (in both freshwater and ocean water), spelunking (caving), climbing, and mountain biking. Swimming in the Segama River was found to be an independent risk factor.[50] With more than 350 imported cases reported from Europe, North and South America, Asia, and Oceania during the past few years, African tick bite fever is currently the most commonly encountered rickettsiosis in travel medicine.[51] Most patients are infected during wild game safaris and bush walks. Moreover, because ecotourism is increasingly popular with international travelers, more cases of imported rickettsioses will likely be seen in the years to come. Cercopithecine herpesvirus 1 (herpes B virus), is an α-herpesvirus endemic in Asian macaques, which mostly carry this virus without overt signs of disease. However, zoonotic infection with herpes B virus in humans usually results in fatal encephalomyelitis or severe neurological impairment.[52] Herpes B virus has been implicated as the cause of approximately forty cases of meningoencephalitis in persons in direct or indirect contact with laboratory macaques. A study was conducted in 105 workers at the Sangeh Monkey Forest in Central Bali to measure contact with macaques (*Macaca fascicularis*) and exposure to herpes B virus. Nearly half of those interviewed had either been bitten or scratched by a macaque, and the prevalence of injury was higher in those who fed macaques. Furthermore, thirty-one of thirty-eight Sangeh macaques had antibodies to herpes B virus. Given that thousands of tourists visit Sangeh during a typical month, a reasonable estimate of the annual number of injuries inflicted by macaques is in the thousands, and Sangeh is but one of a handful of monkey forests on Bali that draw large numbers of visitors.[53]

Petting Zoos and Exotic Pets

Petting zoos, where children are allowed to approach and feed captive wildlife or domestic animals, have been linked to several zoonotic outbreaks, including infections caused by *Escherichia coli* O157:H7, *Salmonella*, and *Coxiella burnetii*.[54–56] More than twenty-five human infectious disease outbreaks were identified during the period 1990–2000 associated with visits to animal exhibits.[54] In an outbreak of *Salmonella* infections at a Colorado zoo, sixty-five cases (most of them in children) were associated with touching a wooden barrier around the Komodo dragon exhibit. *Salmonella* was isolated from thirty-nine case patients, a Komodo dragon, and the wooden barrier. Interestingly, noninfected children were substantially more likely to have washed their hands after visiting the exhibit.[57] Exposure to captive wild animals at circus or zoos can also be a source of zoonotic infection. Twelve circus elephant handlers at an exotic animal farm in Illinois were infected with *M. tuberculosis*, and one handler had signs consistent with active disease after three elephants died of TB. Medical history and testing of the handlers indicated that the elephants had been a probable source of exposure for the majority of the human infections.[26] Seven animal handlers who were previously negative for TB tested positive after a *M. bovis* outbreak in rhinoceroses and monkeys at a zoo in Louisiana.[58] Exotic pets are also a source of several human infections from severe monkeypox related to pet prairie dogs or

Lyssaviruses in pet bats to the less severe but much common ring-worm infections acquired from African pygmy hedgehogs or chin-chillas.[59] Epidemiological and animal traceback investigations confirmed that the first community-acquired human cases of mon-keypox in the United States (seventy-one human cases) resulted from contact with infected prairie dogs that had been housed or transported with African rodents imported from Ghana.[60] Simi-larly, an outbreak caused by *Francisella tularensis* type B occurred among wild-caught, commercially traded prairie dogs, with the presence of *F. tularensis* antibodies in one exposed person the first evidence of prairie dog-to-human tularemia transmission.[61] Lep-tospirosis was diagnosed in two patients exposed at an exotic pet importer company to southern flying squirrels imported from the United States into Japan. *Leptospira* isolates from one patient and five of ten squirrels at the company were genetically and serologi-cally identical and were identified as *Leptospira kirschneri.*[62]

The African pygmy hedgehog has been clearly implicated in human salmonellosis in the United States and Canada. For instance, in Canada, during the period 1994–1996, an increase in the num-ber of laboratory-confirmed cases of human salmonellosis associ-ated with exposure to exotic pets, including iguanas, pet turtles, sugar gliders, and hedgehogs, was observed.[63] In Canada, where about 20,000 laboratory-confirmed annual cases of human salmo-nellosis are reported, 3 to 5 percent of these cases could be asso-ciated to reptile or amphibian exposure.[64] In the United States, the number of commercialized reptiles, especially iguanas, has increased considerably in recent years to reach almost 1 million imported animals per year. The number of human cases of salmo-nellosis, especially in very young children, has also increased dra-matically, in parallel with iguana pet ownership. The Centers for Disease Control and Prevention (CDC) estimate that about 7 per-cent of human *Salmonella* infections in the United States (about 40,000 laboratory confirmed annual cases) are associated with han-dling a reptile. It has been shown that most iguanas have a stable mixture of *Salmonella* serotypes in their intestinal tracts and inter-mittently or continuously shed *Salmonella* organisms in their feces.[65]

Eight cases of rabies, caused by a new rabies virus variant, were reported in the state of Ceará, Brazil, from 1991 to 1998. The marmoset, *Callithrix jacchus*, was determined to be the source of exposure. These primates are commonly used as pets, and most cases occurred in people trying to capture them and in one instance from a pet marmoset.[66] In 1999, an Egyptian rousette (*Rousettus egyptiacus*), imported from Belgium and sold in a pet shop in southwestern France, was diagnosed with encephalitis.[67] This bat was infected with a Lagos bat Lyssavirus, which led to 120 rabies postexposure treatments in people exposed to the pet bat.

Conclusion

Emerging infectious diseases have a major impact on human health and can create a tremendous economic burden.[68] This is well illustrated by the hundreds of millions of dollars in costs associated with the recent epidemic of SARS or H5N1 avian influenza. Animals, particularly wild animals, are thought to be the source of more than 70 percent of all emerging infections.[68] It is therefore essential to develop programs for surveillance and monitoring of emerging diseases in the wildlife reservoir. Two different and complementary approaches have emerged: to monitor the presence of specifically identified pathogens that have emerged as human pathogens, such as Nipah virus, SARS coronavirus, monkeypox virus, Hantaviruses, and prion particles; and to investigate in a given wildlife species the presence of known or unknown viruses and bacteria. For instance, serosurveys of zoonotic agents in various wildlife populations are useful to determine the prevalence rates of zoonotic infections in given regions, such as in free-ranging black and grizzly bears from Alaska or pumas and bobcats from the Americas.[69,70] As suggested by Kuiken and colleagues,[68] it is time to set "a joint expert working group to design and implement a global animal surveillance system for zoonotic pathogens that gives early warning of pathogen emergence, is closely integrated to public health surveillance and provides opportunities to control such pathogens before they can affect human health, food supply, economics or biodiversity."

Better integration and coordination of national surveillance systems are required in both developed and developing countries.[19] Similarly, improved reporting systems and international sharing of information are needed. Active surveillance appears to be essential at the interface of rural populations and wildlife habitats, especially in regions where poverty and low income are increasing the risks of pathogen transmission, as illustrated by the outbreaks of Nipah virus in Bengladesh.[71] Finally, training of professionals, such as veterinarians and biologists in wildlife health management, and establishment of collaborative multidisciplinary teams ready to intervene when outbreaks occur are major tasks that should be undertaken by the international community.[72]

An earlier version of this chapter appeared in *Emerging Infectious Diseases* 13 (2007): 6–11.

References

1. F. R. Lashley (2003), "Factors Contributing to the Occurrence of Emerging Infectious Diseases," *Biological Research for Nursing* 4: 258–67.
2. L. H. Taylor, S. M. Latham, and M. E. Woolhouse (2001), "Risk Factors for Human Disease Emergence," *Philosophical Transactions of the Royal Society of London B: Biological Sciences* 356: 983–89.
3. S. Cleaveland, M. K. Laurenson, and L. H. Taylor (2001), "Diseases of Humans and Their Domestic Mammals: Pathogen Characteristics, Host Range and the Risk of Emergence," *Philosophical Transactions of the Royal Society of London B: Biological Sciences* 356: 991–99.
4. R. G. Bengis, F. A. Leighton, J. R. Fischer, M. Artois, T. Morner, and C. M. Tate (2004), "The Role of Wildlife in Emerging and Re-Emerging Zoonoses," *Revue Scientifique et Technique de l'Office International des Epizooties* 23: 497–511.
5. J. McNeely, K. Miller, W. Reid, R. Mittermeier, and T. Wener (1990), *Conserving the World's Biological Diversity* (Gland, Switzerland: International Union for the Conservation of Nature and Natural Resources; Washington, D.C.: World Resources Institute, Conservation International, World Wildlife Fund-U.S., World Bank).
6. P. Chardonnet, B. des Clers, J. Fisher, R. Gerhold, F. Jori, and F. Lamarque (2002), "The Value of Wildlife," *Revue Scientifique et Technique de l'Office International des Epizooties* 21: 15–51.
7. W. B. Karesh, R. A. Cook, E. L. Bennett, and J. Newcomb (2005), "Wildlife Trade and Global Disease Emergence," *Emerging Infectious Disease* 11: 1000–1002.

8. C. Brown (2004), "Emerging Zoonoses and Pathogens of Public Health Significance: An Overview," *Revue Scientifique et Technique de l'Office International des Epizooties* 23: 435–42.

9. C. D. Harvell, C. E. Mitchell, J. R. Ward, S. Altizer, A. P. Dobson, R. S. Ostfeld, and M. D. Samuel (2002), "Climate Warming and Disease Risks for Terrestrial and Marine Biota," *Science* 296: 2158–62.

10. M. Batista-da-Costa, R. F. Bonito, and S. A. Nishioka (1993), "An Outbreak of Vampire Bat Bite in a Brazilian Village," *Tropical Medicine and Parasitology* 44: 219–20.

11. A. Lopez, P. Miranda, E. Tejada, and D. B. Fishbein (1992), "Outbreak of Human Rabies in the Peruvian Jungle," *Lancet* 339, no. 8790: 408–11.

12. M. C. Schneider, J. Aron, C. Santos-Burgoa, W. Uieda, and S. Ruiz-Velazco (2001), "Common Vampire Bat Attacks on Humans in a Village of the Amazon Region of Brazil," *Cadernos de Saúde Pública* 17: 1531–36.

13. M. C. Schneider, A. Belotto, M. P. Ade, L. F. Leanes, E. Correa, H. Tamayo, G. Medina, and M.G. Rodigues (2005), "Epidemiologic Situation of Human Rabies in Latin America in 2004," *Epidemiological Bulletin* 26: 2–4.

14. M. C. Schneider, C. Santos-Burgoa, J. Aron, B. Munoz, S. Ruiz-Velazco, and W. Uieda (1996), "Potential Force of Infection of Human Rabies Transmitted by Vampire Bats in the Amazonian Region of Brazil," *American Journal of Tropical Medicine and Hygiene* 55: 680–84.

15. C. K. Warner, S. R. Zaki, W. J. Shieh, S. G. Whitfield, J. S. Smith, L. A. Ociari, J. H. Shaddock, M. Niezgoda, C. W. Wright, C. S. Goldsmith, D. W. Sanderlin, P. A. Yager, and C. E. Rupprecht (1999), "Laboratory Investigation of Human Deaths from Vampire Bat Rabies in Peru," *American Journal of Tropical Medicine and Hygiene* 60: 502–7.

16. P. Parola, B. Davoust, and D. Raoult (2005), "Tick- and Flea-Borne Rickettsial Emerging Zoonoses," *Veterinary Research* 36: 469–92.

17. M. G. R. Varma (2001), "Kyasanur Forest Disease," in *The Encyclopedia of Arthropod-Transmitted Infections*, ed. M. W. Service, CABI (London: Oxford University Press), 254–60.

18. M. E. Wise, F. J. Sorvillo, S. C. Shafir, L. R. Ash, and O. G. Berlin (2005), "Severe and Fatal Central Nervous System Disease in Humans Caused by *Baylisascaris procyonis*, the Common Roundworm of Raccoons: A Review of Current Literature," *Microbes and Infection* 7: 317–23.

19. H. Kruse, A. M. Kirkemo, and K. Handeland (2004), "Wildlife as Source of Zoonotic Infections," *Emerging Infectious Diseases* 10: 2067–72.

20. D. H. Walker, A. G. Barbour, J. H. Oliver, R. S. Lane, J. S. Dumler, D. T. Dennis, D. H. Persing, A. F. Azad, and E. McSweegan (1996), "Emerging Bacterial Zoonotic and Vector-Borne Diseases: Ecological and Epidemiological Factors," *Journal of the American Medical Association* 275: 463–69.

21. V. F. Nettles (1992), "Wildlife Diseases and Population Medicine," *Journal of the American Veterinary Medical Association* 200: 648–52.

22. G. P. Roussere, W. J. Murray, C. B. Raudenbush, M. J. Kutilek, D. J. Levee, and K. R. Kazacos (2003), "Raccoon Roundworm Eggs near Homes

and Risk for Larva Migrans Disease, California Communities," *Emerging Infectious Diseases* 9: 1516–22.

23. L. Polley (2005), "Navigating Parasite Webs and Parasite Flow: Emerging and Re-Emerging Parasitic Zoonoses of Wildlife Origin," *International Journal for Parasitology* 35: 1279–94.

24. K. A. Alexander, E. Pleydell, M. C. Williams, E. P. Lane, J. F. Nyange, and A. L. Michel (2002), "*Mycobacterium tuberculosis*: An Emerging Disease of Free-Ranging Wildlife," *Emerging Infectious Diseases* 8: 598–601.

25. S. S. Lewerin, S. L. Olsson, K. Eld, B. Roken, S. Ghebremichael, T. Koivula, G. Kallenius, and G. Bolske (2005), "Outbreak of *Mycobacterium tuberculosis* Infection Among Captive Asian Elephants in a Swedish Zoo," *Veterinary Record* 156: 171–75.

26. K. Michalak, C. Austin, S. Diesel, M. J. Bacon, P. Zimmerman, and J. N. Maslow (1998): *Mycobacterium tuberculosis* Infection as a Zoonotic Disease: Transmission Between Humans and Elephants," *Emerging Infectious Diseases* 4: 283–87.

27. C. J. Phillips, C. R. Foster, P. A. Morris, and R. Teverson (2003), "The Transmission of *Mycobacterium bovis* Infection to Cattle," *Research in Veterinary Science* 74: 1–15.

28. S. M. Schmitt, D. J. O'Brien, C. S. Bruning-Fann, S. D. Fitzgerald (2002), "Bovine Tuberculosis in Michigan Wildlife and Livestock," *Annals of the New York Academy of Science* 969: 262–68.

29. J. Godfroid, A. Cloeckaert, J. P. Liautard, S. Kohler, D. Fretin, and K. Walravens (2005), "From the Discovery of the Malta Fever's Agent to the Discovery of a Marine Mammal Reservoir, Brucellosis Has Continuously Been a Re-emerging Zoonosis," *Veterinary Research* 36: 313–26.

30. J. Godfroid and A. Kasbohrer (2002), "Brucellosis in the European Union and Norway at the Turn of the Twenty-First Century," *Veterinary Microbiology* 90: 135–45.

31. P. Daszak, A. A. Cunningham, and A. D. Hyatt (2001), "Anthropogenic Environmental Change and the Emergence of Infectious Diseases in Wildlife," *Acta Tropica* 78: 103–16.

32. P. R. Wilson (2002), "Advances in Health and Welfare of Farmed Deer in New Zealand," *New Zealand Veterinary Journal* 50, no. 3 (Suppl): 105–9.

33. R. S. Veazey, C. C. Vice, D. Y. Cho, T. N. Tully, Jr., and S. M. Shane (1994), "Pathology of Eastern Equine Encephalitis in Emus (*Dromaius novaehollandiae*)," *Veterinary Pathology* 31: 109–11.

34. S. E. Sanford (1995), "Outbreaks of Yersiniosis Caused by *Yersinia pseudotuberculosis* in Farmed Cervids," *Journal of Veterinary Diagnostic Investigation* 7: 78–81.

35. E. Check (2004), "Health Concerns Prompt U.S. Review of Exotic-Pet Trade," *Nature* 427: 277.

36. M. H. Woodford and P. B. Rossiter (1993), "Disease Risks Associated with Wildlife Translocation Projects," *Revue Scientifique et Technique de l'Office International des Epizooties* 12: 115–35.

37. G. W. Lee, K. A. Lee, and W. R. Davidson (1993), "Evaluation of Fox-Chasing Enclosures as Sites of Potential Introduction and Estab-

lishment of *Echinococcus multilocularis,*" *Journal of Wildlife Diseases* 29: 498–501.

38. D. G. Constantine (2003), "Geographic Translocation of Bats: Known and Potential Problems," *Emerging Infectious Diseases* 9: 17–21.

39. K. De Schrijver (1998), "A Psittacosis Outbreak in Customs Officers in Antwerp (Belgium)," *Bulletin of the Institute of Maritime and Tropical Medicine in Gdynia* 49: 97–99.

40. S. Van Borm, I. Thomas, G. Hanquet, B. Lambrecht, M. Boschmans, G. Dupont, M. Decaestecker, R. Snacken, and T. van den Berg (2005), "Highly Pathogenic H5N1 Influenza Virus in Smuggled Thai Eagles, Belgium," *Emerging Infectious Diseases* 11: 702–5.

41. N. D. Wolfe, W. Heneine, J. K. Carr, A. D. Garcia, Vedapuri Shanmugam, U. Tamoufe, J. N. Torimiro, A. T. Prosser, M. LeBreton, E. Mpoudi-Ngole, F. E. McCutchan, D. L. Birx, T. M. Folks, D. S. Burke, and W. M. Switzer (2005), "Emergence of Unique Primate T-Lymphotropic Viruses Among Central African Bushmeat Hunters," *Proceedings of the National Academy of Science* 102: 7994–99.

42. B. M. Kuehn (2005), "New Human Retroviruses Discovered: Evidence That Cross-Species Leap Not a Rare Event," *Journal of the American Medical Association* 293: 2989–90.

43. M. C. Georges-Courbot, A. Sanchez, C. Y. Lu, S. Baize, E. Leroy, J. Lansout-Soukate, C. Tevi-Benissan, A. J. Georges, S. G. Trappier, S. R. Zaki, R. Swanepoel, P. A. Leman, P. E. Rollin, C. J. Peters, S. T. Nichol, and T. G. Ksiazek (1997), "Isolation and Phylogenetic Characterization of Ebola Viruses Causing Different Outbreaks in Gabon," *Emerging Infectious Diseases* 3: 59–62.

44. F. Hayden and A. Croisier (2005), "Transmission of Avian Influenza Viruses to and Between Humans," *Journal of Infectious Disease* 192: 1311–14.

45. P. Daszak, G. M. Tabor, A. M. Kilpatrick, J. Epstein, and R. Plowright (2004), "Conservation Medicine and a New Agenda for Emerging Diseases," *Annals of the New York Academy of Science* 1026: 1–11.

46. S. K. P. Lau, P. C. Y. Woo, K. S. M. Li, Y. Huang, H-W. Tsoi, B. H. L. Wong, S. S. Y. Wong, S-Y. Leung, K.-H. Chan, and K.-Y. Yuen (2005), "Severe Acute Respiratory Syndrome Coronavirus-Like Virus in Chinese Horseshoe Bats," *Proceedings of the National Academy of Science* 102: 14040–45.

47. Centers for Disease Control and Prevention (2004), "Trichinellosis Associated with Bear Meat—New York and Tennessee, 2003," *Morbidity and Mortality Weekly Report* 53: 606–10.

48 K. Takahashi, N. Kitajima, N. Abe, and S. Mishiro (2004), "Complete or Near-Complete Nucleotide Sequences of Hepatitis E Virus Genome Recovered From a Wild Boar, a Deer, and Four Patients Who Ate the Deer," *Virology* 330: 501–5.

49. C. N. Macpherson (2005), "Human Behaviour and the Epidemiology of Parasitic Zoonoses," *International Journal for Parasitology* 35: 1319–31.

50. J. Sejvar, E. Bancroft, K. Winthrop, J. Bettinger, M. Bajani, S. Bragg, K. Shutt, R. Kaiser, N. Marano, T. Popovic, J. Tappero, D. Ashford, L. Mascola, D. Vugia, D. Perkins, and N. Rosenstein (2003), "Leptospirosis in 'Eco-Challenge' Athletes, Malaysian Borneo, 2000," *Emerging Infectious Disease* 9: 702–7.

51. M. Jensenius, P. E. Fournier, and D. Raoult (2004), "Rickettsioses and the International Traveler," *Clinical Infectious Disease* 39: 1493–99.

52. J. L. Huff and P. A. Barry (2003), "B-Virus (Cercopithecine Herpesvirus 1) Infection in Humans and Macaques: Potential for Zoonotic Disease," *Emerging Infectious Disease* 9: 246–50.

53. G. A. Engel, L. Jones-Engel, M. A. Schillaci, K. G. Suaryana, A. Putra, A. Fuentes, and R. Henkel (2002), "Human Exposure to Herpesvirus B-Seropositive Macaques, Bali, Indonesia," *Emerging Infectious Disease* 8: 789–95.

54. J. B. Bender and S. A. Shulman (2004), "Reports of zoonotic disease outbreaks associated with animal exhibits and availability of recommendations for preventing zoonotic disease transmission from animals to people in such settings," *Journal of the American Veterinary Medical Association* 224: 1105–9.

55. Centers for Disease Control and Prevention (2005), "Outbreaks of *Escherichia coli* O157:H7 Associated with Petting Zoos—North Carolina, Florida, and Arizona, 2004 and 2005," *Morbidity and Mortality Weekly Report* 54:1277–1280.

56. Tissot-Dupont H, Amadei MA, Nezri M, Raoult D. (2005), "A pedagogical farm as a source of q Fever in a French city," *European Journal of Epidemiology* 20: 957–61.

57. C. R. Friedman, C. Torigian, P. L. Shillam, R. E. Hoffman, D. Heltzel, J. L. Beebe, G. Malcolm, W. E. DeWitt, L. Hutwagner, and P. M. Griffin (1998), "An Outbreak of Salmonellosis Among Children Attending a Reptile Exhibit at a Zoo," *Journal of Pediatrics* 132: 802–7.

58. Stetter MD, Mikota SK, Gutter AF, Monterroso ER, Dalovisio JR, Degraw C, Farley (1995), "Epizootic of *Mycobacterium bovis* in a Zoologic Park," *Journal of the American Veterinary Medical Association* 207: 1618–21.

59. T. Rosen and J. Jablon (2003), "Infectious Threats from Exotic Pets: Dermatological Implications," *Dermatology Clinics* 21: 229–36.

60. Centers for Disease Control and Prevention (2003), "Update: Multistate Outbreak of Monkeypox—Illinois, Indiana, Kansas, Missouri, Ohio, and Wisconsin, 2003," *Morbidity and Mortality Weekly Report* 52: 642–46.

61. S. B. Avashia, J. M. Petersen, C. M. Lindley, M. E. Schriefer, K. L. Gage, M. Cetron, T. A. DeMarcus, D. K. Kim, J. Buck, J. A. Montenieri, J. L. Lowell, M. F. Antolin, M. Y. Kosoy, L. G. Carter, M. C. Chu, K. A. Hendricks, D. T. Dennis, and J. L. Kool (2004), "First Reported Prairie Dog-to-Human Tularemia Transmission, Texas, 2002," *Emerging Infectious Disease* 10: 483–86.

62. T. Masuzawa, Y. Okamoto, Y. Une, T. Takeuchi, K. Tsukagoshi, N. Koizumi, H. Kawabata, S. Ohta, and Y. Yoshikawa Y. (2006), "Leptospirosis

in Squirrels Imported from United States to Japan," *Emerging Infectious Diseases* 12: 1153–55.

63. P. Y. Riley and B. B. Chomel (2005), "Hedgehog Zoonoses," *Emerging Infectious Diseases* 11: 1–5.

64. D. L. Woodward, R. Khakhria, and W. M. Johnson (1997), "Human Salmonellosis Associated with Exotic Pets," *Journal of Clinical Microbiology* 35: 2786–90.

65. B. R. Burnham, D. H. Atchley, R. P. DeFusco, K. E. Ferris, J. C. Zicarelli, J, H. Lee, and F. J. Angulo (1998), "Prevalence of Fecal Shedding of *Salmonella* Organisms Among Captive Green Iguanas and Potential Public Health Implications," *Journal of the American Veterinary Medical Association* 213: 48–50.

66. S. R. Favoretto, C. C. de Mattos, N. B. Morais, F. A. Alves Araujo, and C. A. de Mattos (2001), "Rabies in Marmosets (*Callithrix jacchus*), Ceara, Brazil," *Emerging Infectious Diseases* 7: 1062–65.

67. Y. Rotivel, M. Goudal, H. Bourhy, and H. Tsiang (2001), "La rage des chiroptères en France, 2001: Actualités et importance en santé publique," *Bulletin Epidemiologique et Hebdomadaire* 39 (September 23), http://www.invs.sante.fr/beh (accessed November 22, 2006).

68. T. Kuiken, F. A. Leighton, R. A. Fouchier, J. W. Leduc, J. S. M. Peiris, A. Schudel, and K. Stohr (2005), "Public Health: Pathogen Surveillance in Animals," *Science* 309: 1680–81.

69. B. B. Chomel, R. W. Kasten, G. Chappuis, M. Soulier, and Y. Kikuchi (1998), "Serological Survey of Selected Canine Viral Pathogens and Zoonoses in Grizzly Bears (*Ursus arctos horribilis*) and Black Bears (*Ursus americanus*) from Alaska," *Revue Scientifique et Technique de l'Office International des Epizooties* 17: 756–66.

70. B. B. Chomel, Y. Kikuchi, J. S. Martenson, M. E. Roelke-Parker, C. Chang, R. W. Kasten, J. E. Foley, J. Laudre, K. Murphy, P. K. Swift, V. L. Kramer, and S. J. O'Brien (2004), "Seroprevalence of *Bartonella* Infection in American Free-ranging and Captive Pumas (*Felis concolor*) and Bobcats (*Lynx rufus*)," *Veterinary Research* 35: 233–41.

71. World Health Organization (2004), "Nipah Virus Outbreak(s) in Bangladesh-January-April 2004," *Weekly Epidemiological Record* 79: 168–71.

72. B. B. Chomel, A. Belotto, and F.-X. Meslin (2007), "Wildlife, Exotic Pets, and Emerging Zoonoses," *Emerging Infectious Diseases* 13: 6–11.

Chapter 12
Monkeypox
A Threat to the United States?

Darin S. Carroll

This chapter deals primarily with ecological studies of the genus *Orthopoxvirus monkeypox*, which is associated with a febrile rash zoonotic disease in humans. Compared to other zoonoses, relatively little is known regarding the ecology and natural history of this species. What is known indicates that rodents likely serve as the reservoir host(s) of monkeypox. For this chapter a reservoir is defined as a population or group of populations that are epidemiologically linked and that serve as a permanent source of infection for the population of interest (as modified from Haydon et al.).[1] In this context, the population of interest is the human population. In many zoonotic disease systems, humans are dead-end hosts and play no role in the maintenance of the disease in nature. Thus, to really understand the disease, it is important to examine the interaction between the pathogen and its reservoir hosts. An example of the importance of this can be found in a case study of Bolivian hemorrhagic fever, which is caused by the Machupo virus (a member of the Family Arenaviridae).[2] The rodent reservoir of this infection is the Large Vesper mouse, *Calomys callosus*. This species is broadly distributed, from northern Bolivia south to central Argentina. Nevertheless, human cases of Bolivian hemorrhagic fever have been identified only in northern Bolivia. Early on, this distribution of human cases confused researchers, given the distribution of the rodent host. However, although the mouse in northern Bolivia looks very similar to the mouse in central Argentina, genetic profiling shows several genetically distinct populations scattered throughout the range of what is called one species. The population of *C. callosus* that occurs in the disease endemic area of Bolivian hemorrhagic fever is genetically distinct from all the other *Calomys* populations and thus seems to be the real reservoir host of the virus, which explains the disease's limited range.

Poxviruses

Most of the highly pathogenic poxviruses belong to the genus *Orthopoxvirus*.[3] The most famous members of this genus are variola, the causative agent of smallpox, and vaccinia, a virus closely related to the cowpox virus—and the platform for several vaccines. Current data suggest that most orthopoxviruses persist in rodent reservoirs. Additionally, it seems likely that variola virus (or its progenitor) was once an infection of rodents that somehow made the jump into humans and became exclusively associated with them. The eradication of smallpox was facilitated by this exclusive association with a single host. It is important to note that the eradication effort would not likely have been possible if there had been an animal reservoir. The eradication of smallpox has left monkeypox as the most severe extant *Orthopoxvirus* in terms of the severity of the resultant disease.

Monkeypox

Monkeypox is endemic to the Congo Basin area and sub-Saharan Africa, but in 2003 it infected people in the Midwestern United States—the first report of human infections outside Africa. That is not the first time the virus was found in the United States. There have been cases in animals, mostly in laboratory colonies of primates that were collected in Africa and then sent to research labs in Europe and the United States. This is the origin of the name monkeypox (which is unfortunate, because nonhuman primates, like humans, are almost certainly dead-end hosts that do not play a role in maintenance of the disease in the wild). Human monkeypox was not identified until near the end of the smallpox eradication program in Africa (in 1970). Surveillance efforts found cases that looked similar to smallpox in areas previously covered by the eradication campaign. Initially, it was thought that the eradication effort had missed these cases, but they were identified as human monkeypox. Human monkeypox causes a rashlike illness almost indistinguishable clinically from smallpox. However, the average case fatality rate for monkeypox (up to 10 percent) is usually less than that for smallpox, and monkeypox patients have distinct lymphadenopathy, which is not typical of smallpox. Additionally, monkeypox has only limited human-to-human transmission, whereas smallpox is fairly efficient. The longest documented chain of human-to-human transmission for monkeypox is six transmission events (documented in 2003 in the Republic of Congo). Nevertheless, the similarities between the two diseases are sufficient to be a cause for concern, especially if monkeypox were to become more efficient in terms of person-to-person transmission.

Monkeypox in the United States

The monkeypox virus that was introduced into the United States in 2003 arrived in a shipment of animals from Ghana. Ironically, there has never been a documented human monkeypox case from Ghana. Nevertheless, the Ghanaian government was extremely helpful in facilitating the CDC investigation that followed this introduction into the United States. It was subsequently determined that hundreds of rodents had been collected in Ghana, shipped in the belly of a commercial jetliner to a dealer in Texas, and then transferred to a dealer in Illinois. At some point these African rodents came in contact with North American rodents (black-tailed prairie dogs, *Cynomys ludovicianus*), which are easily infected with monkeypox. The virus was then transmitted to people in Midwestern states from these prairie dogs. Many of the imported African rodents died, but it was difficult to decide how many had died from monkeypox and how many because of the shipping conditions The prairie dogs certainly showed a much more dramatic disease than did the African animals, and, as unfortunate as that outbreak was, the CDC learned a great deal regarding the natural history of the disease.

First, genomic sequencing showed the existence of two monkeypox clades (Congo Basin and the West African), with significant differences in the epidemiological and clinical features of the resultant human disease caused by each member of the clade. The Congo Basin human monkeypox disease is characterized by a more pronounced morbidity, mortality, and human-to-human transmission than is seen in the human disease caused by West African–derived virus (the virus that caused disease in the United States).[4] It also became obvious that many other orthopoxviruses likely exist, all of which are cross-reactive with the antibody assays originally used to identify monkeypox virus infection.

Could Monkeypox Become Established in the United States?

It remains to be determined whether monkeypox could become established in the United States, either as the result of transmission to native North American species or through the introduction of an infected invasive reservoir host from Africa (for example, a population of African pouched rats has recently become established in the Florida Keys, although none of the animals examined has shown evidence of infection with monkeypox virus). Following the human monkeypox outbreak in the United States, animal specimens were submitted to the CDC by state departments of health and agriculture for evaluation. These included animals involved directly in the shipment from Ghana, animals associated with people with monkeypox, and animals from the exotic animal dealership in Illinois suspected to have been the site of monkeypox transmission from imported African rodents to North American prairie dogs. Sixteen species showed evidence of infection.[5] However, a further collaborative study between the U.S. Department of Agriculture (USDA) Wildlife Services and the U.S. Geological Survey's National Wildlife Health Center (NWHC) found no evidence of monkeypox virus infection in putative reservoir species wild caught in the area of the 2003 outbreak in the United States. Similar studies in Illinois also failed to find any evidence of establishment.[5]

What Are the Reservoir Hosts in Africa?

To date, the reservoir species (one or more) of monkeypox virus remain undetermined. Two approaches have been used. In the first, various species of African rodents and primates are investigated directly for evidence of infection. In the second, the distribution of human disease and the distribution of putative animal hosts are compared.

Three of the African rodent species in the shipment to Texas (giant pouched rats, *Cricetomys* spp.; rope squirrels, *Funisciurus* sp.; and dormice, *Graphiurus* sp.) were monkeypox virus positive, but it was not known for certain which species introduced the infection into the crate and which had become infected during transit.[5] The investigation continued in Ghana, where CDC investigators met with the people who collected the rodents and visited the locations where the rodents were collected (the Ghanaian collectors used old soup cans with a sock at one end to trap rodents driven from their burrows by smoke from a small fire). Wild-caught examples of all three species of rodents that were infected in the shipment crate turned out to be virus positive. However, previous studies had provided long lists of captive and wild-caught primates and rodents (and other mammals) that showed some (good or bad) evidence of infection with monkeypox virus.[6] Evidence of infection or exposure alone is not evidence that the species in question is the reservoir host. Because much more is known about the distribution of human monkeypox than about the natural sylvatic cycles of this virus in nonhuman animal hosts, simply overlaying human monkeypox case data from Africa on the known or suspected distribution of putative reservoir hosts could be used to rule out or justify the further investigation of a particular species. One of the squirrels mentioned in some of the earlier literature as being important in the transmission of monkeypox can be ruled out in just this way. In fact, this comparison of distributions led back to a shorter species list that includes all three (giant pouched rats, *Cricetomys* spp.; rope squirrels, *Funisciuris* sp.; and dormice, *Graphiurus* sp.) that were infected in the U.S. shipment. Unfortunately, the taxonomy of these rodents is far from certain and, remembering the example of Bolivian hemorrhagic fever that opened this chapter, it would be premature to drawn any hard-and-fast conclusions. For example, the giant pouched rat, *Cricetomys* spp., is often reported in the popular press to be the reservoir of the monkeypox virus. Prior to the CDC investigation in Ghana, it was believed there were two species of giant pouched rat, but as a result of our investigation it is thought that there may be at least four and possibly more. It will be some time before the reservoir host species can be definitely identified.[7]

Next Steps

In response to the 2003 outbreak in the United States, the following steps were taken to prevent monkeypox from being re-introduced or established in the country.

The CDC Web page on monkeypox contained the statement:

On June 11, 2003, the Centers for Disease Control and Prevention (CDC) and the Food and Drug Administration (FDA) issued a joint order prohibiting the importation of all African rodents into the United States. The joint order also banned within the United States any sale, offering for distribution, transport, or release into the environment, of prairie dogs and six specific genera of African rodents. The joint order was enacted as part of the public health response to the first reported outbreak of monkeypox in the United States. On November 4, 2003, the joint order was replaced by an interim final rule which maintains the bans on importation of African rodents and the sale, distribution, transport, and release into the environment as previously described. Currently, a person may not import into the United States any rodent of African origin, including any rodents that were caught in Africa and then shipped directly to the United States or shipped to other countries before being imported to the United States. The prohibition also applies to rodents whose native habitat is in Africa, even if those rodents were born elsewhere. These animals may still be imported for scientific, exhibition, or educational purposes with a valid permit issued by CDC.

This prohibition was based on the best scientific evidence available, but, as the foregoing sections make clear, the actual reservoir host species of monkeypox virus is still unknown. Nor is identification likely to be easy. Animals are imported across national borders (legally and illegally) all the time (see Chapter 6). Zoonotic disease agents can and have been translocated thousands of miles from regions where they exist in endemic sylvatic cycles. The introduction of monkeypox into human populations in the United States in 2003 reminds us how easily globalization can cause a breach in the ecological compartmentalization (see Chapter 10) that tends to keep us safe."

The findings and conclusions in this report are those of the author and do not necessarily represent the views of the Centers for Disease Control and Prevention or the U.S. government.

References

1. D. T. Haydon, S. Cleaveland, L. H. Taylor, and M. K. Laurenson (2002), "Identifying Reservoirs of Infection: A Conceptual and Practical Challenge." *Emerging Infectious Diseases* 8: 1468–73.

2. P. E. Kilgore, C. J. Peters, J. N. Mills, P. E. Rollin, L. Armstrong, A. S. Khan, and T. G. Ksiazek (1995), "Prospects for the Control of Bolivian Hemorrhagic Fever," *Emerging Infectious Diseases* 1: 97–100.

3. P. D. Acha and B. Szyfres (2003), *Zoonoses and Communicable Diseases Common to Man and Animals*, 3rd ed., vol. II, *Chlamydioses, Rickettsioses and Viroses*, Scientific and Technical Publication No. 580 (Pan American Health Organization), 84–88.

4. A. M. Likos, S. A. Sammons, V. A. Olson, A. M. Frace, Y. Li, M. Olsen-Rasmussen, et al. (2005), "A Tale of Two Clades: Monkeypox Viruses," *Journal of General Virology* 86: 2661–72.

5. C. L. Hutson, K. N. Lee, J. Abel, D. S. Carroll, J. M. Montgomery, V.A. Olson, Y. Li, W. Davidson, C. Hughes, M. Dillon, P. Spurlock, J. J. Kazmierczak, A. Austin, L. Miser, F. E.Sorhage, J. Howell, J. P. Davis, M. G. Reynolds, Z. Braden, K. L. Karem, I. K. Damon, and R. L. Regnery (2007), "Monkeypox Zoonotic Associations: Insights from Laboratory Evaluation of Animals Associated with the Multi-state US Outbreak," *American Journal of Tropical Medicine and Hygiene* 76: 757–67.

6. A. J. Robinson and P. J. Kerr (2001), "Poxvirus Infections," in *Infectious Diseases of Wild Mammals*, 3rd ed., ed. E. S. Williams and I. K. Barker (London: Manson Publishing, Veterinary Press), 179–201.

7. Lynne A. Learned, Mary G. Reynolds, Demole Wassa Wassa, Yu Li, Victoria A. Olson, Kevin Karem, Linda L. Stempora, Zach H. Braden, Richard Kline, Anna Likos, François Libama, Henri Moudzeo, Jean Daniel Bolanda, Paul Tarangonia, Paul Boumandoki, Pierre Formenty, Joseph M. Harvey, and Inger K. Damon (2005), "Extended Interhuman Transmission of Monkeypox in a Hospital Community in the Republic of the Congo, 2003," *American Journal of Tropical Medicine and Hygiene* 73:2: 428–434.

Chapter 13
Bat Zoonoses
The Realities

Charles Rupprecht, Lin-Fa Wang, and Leslie A. Real

Bats may be the most "abundant, diverse, and geographically dispersed" of all vertebrates.[1] Twenty percent of all mammalian species are bats. They feed on insects, mammals, fishes, blood, fruit, and pollen and are found on all continents except Antarctica. These remarkable animals are increasingly recognized as reservoir hosts for viruses that can cross species barriers to infect humans and other domestic and wild mammals. In the rabies literature, this crossing of species barriers is referred to as "spillover." Bats evolved early, and it has been suggested that the capacity for spillover manifested by some of the viruses maintained in bats may be explained by a long history of co-speciation, in which viral replication depended on cellular receptors and biochemical pathways that are conserved in mammals that evolved later.[1] Bats have been found to be infected with viruses from at least eighteen viral families; they are known to be reservoirs for Lyssaviruses and for Nipah and Hendra viruses, and they may well be the reservoir for the severe acute respiratory syndrome (SARS) coronavirus and Ebola virus. Messenger and colleagues[2] as well as Calisher and colleagues[1] have summarized the several attributes of the life histories and natural histories of bat species that facilitate their role as reservoir hosts: they are long-lived, they can fly (some species fly many hundreds of miles), their crowded roosting behavior increases the likelihood of intra- and interspecies transmission of viral infections (bats are the most abundant mammal), some Lyssaviruses are transplacentally transmitted in bats, and several of the viruses that are highly pathogenic for humans and other vertebrates are believed to infect and persist in apparently healthy bats.

This chapter deals with two groups of bat viruses. One group, the Lyssaviruses, consists of virus species that have long been known to infect bats (although new representatives are being discovered all the time). The other, which consists of the SARS coronavirus-like viruses, have only recently come to our attention.

Rabies and the Lyssaviruses

Rabies is the quintessential—if not the most important—viral zoonosis. It has the highest case fatality rate of any infectious disease, it is essentially incurable, and, with the exception of Antarctica, it can be found just about everywhere. Rabies is not a rare disease. By the time you finish reading this chapter, at least two people will have died from rabies, and probably one of them was a child. Rabies is caused by a Lyssavirus.

The Origins and Evolution of the Lyssaviruses

Currently, we know of at least seven genotypes of Lyssavirus: the classic rabies virus (genotype 1) and the rabies-related viruses (genotypes 2–7). Four other viruses, Aravan, Khujand, Irkut, and West Caucasian bat virus, may also be genotypes of the Lyssavirus genus.[3]

Insectivorous bats are probable vectors for six of the Lyssavirus genotypes and are exclusive to three of them. Although we habitually think of rabies in terms of infected dogs, cats, and raccoons, Lyssaviruses in general evolved in insectivorous bats (*Chiroptera* spp.) long before they switched hosts and emerged in terrestrial carnivores.[4] It is speculated that Lyssaviruses derive from a plant rhabdovirus. Insectivorous bats became infected with the Lyssavirus progenitor between 7,000 and 12,000 years ago as the result of feeding on insects that were themselves infected with a plant rhabdovirus.[4]

Spillover infections from bat hosts to other mammalian hosts occur quite commonly—indeed, most indigenously acquired cases of human rabies in the United States are the result of exposure to infected bats. However, recent work from the Institut Pasteur suggests that these common spillover events only infrequently resulted in Lyssaviruses becoming established in terrestrial mammals. Phylogenetic analysis suggests that one spillover event resulted in the genotype 1 becoming established in raccoons (and possibly skunks) in North America and a second spillover event resulted in the same genotype becoming established in terrestrial carnivores in the Old World. This second event is thought to have occurred sometime between 888 and 1,459 years ago. The 4,000-year-old accounts of a disease in Mesopotamia that sounds very much like rabies are explained by suggesting that previous spill events from bats to carnivores have occurred but that the translocated Lyssavirus was unable to persist in its new host for sufficiently long to be recognized today. This should not surprise us; modern phylogenetic tools demonstrate that virus lineages become extinct.[4]

The molecular revolution, the expanding use of molecular techniques to study viral evolution and transmission dynamics, has provided us with a much greater understanding of host virus interactions and of the epidemiology of zoonotic disease. It has also drawn our attention to viruses that are of trivial public health significance today but that may become problematic. Traditionally, viruses were classified by serological reactivity. For example, serological distinctions were used to classify Duvenhage virus, Mokola virus, and Lagos bat virus as distinct Lyssavirus serotypes.[5] Modern sequencing techniques showed that this classification was correct. However, serological cross-reactivity studies also placed seven other viruses within the genus Lyssavirus, which sequencing studies have demonstrated was incorrect.[6] Thus, sequencing can be used to assess the degree of relatedness of viruses within and between genera and clearly shows, for example, that the Lyssaviruses recently discovered as the result of active surveillance in bats (Aravan, Khujand, Irkut, and West Caucasian bat virus) are only distantly related to the genotype 1 classic rabies virus. The significance of this is that conventional pre-exposure vaccination or conventional postexposure prophylaxis affords no significant protection against the most genetically divergent of these viruses (West Caucasian bat virus). In short, the propensity of Lyssaviruses to spill over from bat reservoirs and become established in terrestrial mammals means that today's biological curiosities may be tomorrow's translocated headaches.

Globalization, Food, Spillover, and Rabies in the Americas

Many of us who deal with emerging zoonoses hold the view that globalization is not a new phenomenon: it has been going on from the time life evolved and Pangea started breaking up. It has been enhanced for about the last million years or so, and probably exacerbated over the last few centuries. Rabies in the Americas provides a good example.

During the period 1993–2002, the Americas reported an 82 percent decrease in the number of human cases. In 1993 the total number of cases was 216 (mortality rate, 0.03 per 100,000 inhabitants) and in 2002 the number of cases was 39 (mortality rate, <0.01 per 100,000 inhabitants).[7] The elimination of human rabies transmitted by dogs has been a fundamental goal of national and international public health agencies throughout the Americas and is a goal that is approaching fulfillment. Nevertheless, rabies in certain species of wildlife still poses a potential risk to people in every country in the Americas, including North America and many countries of the Caribbean. For example, between 1993 and 2002, bats (various species) were the second most common transmitter of rabies to humans in the Americas, accounting for 14.7 percent (168 cases) of all cases recorded.[7] In Latin America, the majority of human cases in which the bat species was identified involved the hematophagous (vampire) bat (*Desmodus rotundus*). Risk factors for vampire bat attacks on humans in Latin America include the removal of livestock, deforestation, and gold mining;[7] indeed, anthoprogenic factors (including "globalization" in its most limited sense) have long been influential in the history of rabies throughout the Americas.

Rabies in carnivores had been recognized in the Old World for thousands of years; however, most of the earliest explorers remarked on its notable absence in the Americas, at least in dogs, until the early 1700s.[8] Additionally, there is almost no oral or written record from the Meso-American peoples or from Cherokee traditions (for example) of anything like rabies. Currently, by conservative estimates, there are at least thirteen distinct genotype 1 classic rabies Lyssavirus variants in North America. By reconstructing the evolution of the variants in bats in North America it has proved possible to piece together a convincing history of the introduction and spread of rabies in the Americas.

Based on the fossil record, several species of vampire bats were once widely distributed throughout North America. During the Quaternary period, many large-bodied and abundant mammalian species may have served as suitable prey for vampire bats, but these perished during the Pleistocene extinctions, creating a relative shortage in blood supply and a consequent contraction in vampire bat population numbers and distribution. With the colonization of the Americas ("New Spain"), the introduction of cattle should have allowed the local reexpansion of hematophagous bat populations (for example, current *Desmodus* populations are larger in livestock areas of Argentina than in non-cattle-rearing regions). Molecular studies suggest that the ancestor of modern rabies virus variants was introduced from Europe into Middle or South America sometime in the seventeenth century—coinciding with the inferred expansion of vampire bat populations. The descendants of this virus engendered the expanding (nonmigratory) vampire bat populations and also populations of migratory bat species. Once the virus reached bat populations in North America, there was a period of very rapid adaptation to new bat host species, giving rise to the rabies virus variants we see today, including those variants found in terrestrial mammal species.

Spillover from bats and establishment in previously nonadapted hosts continues to this day. For example, rabies had not been detected in terrestrial wildlife in northern Arizona until 2001, when rabies was diagnosed in nineteen rabid skunks in Flagstaff. The virus was not related to viruses found in other terrestrial carnivores; however, it did show monoclonal antibody patterns similar to the rabies viruses found in big brown (*Eptesicus fuscus*) and *Myotis* bats in the western United States. Given that so many skunks were infected, it was thought that the epidemic could be most easily explained by one (or a few) bat-to-skunk transmissions, followed by self-sustaining skunk-to-skunk chains of infection. It is also worth noting that the outbreak occurred in a peri-urban area and that both the big brown bat and *Myotis* commonly roost in buildings.[9]

Rabies Control

We know that the elimination of canine rabies virus is possible.[7] We also know that rabies in wildlife can be controlled and sometimes eliminated. In both cases, the process depends on the availability of an effective vaccine and a practical means of deployment (usually in conjunction with extensive education campaigns and appropriate legislation to ensure compliance with vaccination protocols in domestic animals). The introduction of recombinant oral rabies virus vaccines transformed our ability to control rabies in terrestrial wildlife species and showed promise for domestic species, too.[10,11] But why not think about other means of deployment that might broaden the spectrum of affected wildlife species that could be included in rabies control programs? These other means might include prey items, such as transgenic insects that express rabies virus glycoproteins, or the use of extoparasites as "natural hypodemics."

SARS-like Coronaviruses in Bats

SARS is caused by a coronavirus. Beginning in November 2002 and ending in July 2003, the first SARS pandemic spread to thirty-three countries and involved more than 8,000 infections, with over 700 deaths.[12,13] Sporadic outbreaks later occurred in 2003 and 2004 in the People's Republic of China, but molecular epidemiological studies showed that the SARS coronaviruses responsible for the 2003–2004 outbreaks were not the same as those isolated during the 2002–2003 outbreaks.[12] This suggested that SARS had an animal reservoir and that there had been at least two independent spillover events. Evidence that SARS did in fact have an animal origin accumulated quickly. For example, genome sequencing showed that the SARS coronavirus was a new virus with no genetic relatedness to any known human coronaviruses; there was no evidence of previous exposure to the SARS coronavirus in the human population; serological surveys among market traders during the 2002–2003 outbreaks showed that antibodies against SARS coronavirus were present at a higher ratio in animal traders than in control populations; and SARS coronaviruses isolated from animals in markets were almost identical to human isolates. Initially, palm civets were implicated as a potential reservoir, but the lack of widespread infection in wild or farmed palm civets rendered this conclusion unlikely.

Recently, though, two independently working research groups found SARS-like coronaviruses in different species of horseshoe bats (genus *Rhinolophus*). Sequence analyses showed that the SARS-like coronaviruses found in horseshoe bats manifested a much greater genetic diversity than the SARS coronaviruses isolated from civets or humans. This is good evidence that the virus responsible for SARS in people is a member of this novel coronavirus group and that bats are a natural reservoir for it.[12] However, it should be noted that current studies suggest that the SARS-like coronaviruses found in horseshoe bats would probably not be able to infect people (they are unable to make efficient use of human receptor molecules). In that case a period of rapid viral evolution in an intermediate host (such as a civet) would be necessary to adapt the virus for human infection. Another possibility is that the human SARS coronavirus originated from a bat species yet to be identified. This species may or may not be in China; wildlife trafficking between China and neighboring countries makes it difficult to determine.

Bats and Ebola Virus?

According to the Centers for Disease Control and Prevention,

> Ebola hemorrhagic fever is a severe, often-fatal disease in humans and nonhuman primates (monkeys, gorillas, and chimpanzees) that has appeared sporadically since its initial recognition in 1976. The disease is caused by infection with Ebola virus, named after a river in the Democratic Republic of the Congo (formerly Zaire) in Africa, where it was first recognized. . . . The virus can be transmitted in several ways. People can be exposed to Ebola virus from direct contact with the blood or secretions of an infected person. Thus, the virus is often spread through families and friends because they come in close contact with such secretions when caring for infected persons. People can also be exposed to Ebola virus through contact with objects, such as needles, that have been contaminated with infected secretions. Nosocomial transmission . . . occurs frequently during Ebola outbreaks.[14]

Ebola virus is composed of four known species: Ebola virus Zaire, Ebola virus Sudan, Ebola virus Côte d'Ivoire, and Ebola virus Reston. Ebola virus Zaire occurs in Gabon, the Republic of Congo, and the Democratic Republic of Congo. Between October 2001 and May 2003, five Ebola outbreaks in humans, with a total of 313 cases and 264 deaths, occurred in Gabon and the Republic of Congo. These outbreaks were due to the Ebola virus Zaire subtype, which is the most virulent. Up to 78 percent of the patients died, usually within five to seven days. Great ape populations (gorillas and chimpanzees) in Gabon and the Republic of Congo have also been devastated by Ebola hemorrhagic fever, leaving these two species critically endangered (great ape density is estimated to have fallen by 180 percent over the past decade).[15]

Recently, Leroy and colleagues[16] presented compelling evidence that three species of fruit bats, *Hypsignathus monstrosus*, *Epomops franqueti*, and *Myonycteris torquata*, may constitute a wildlife reservoir for Ebola virus Zaire. These bats, which can be trapped near the villages affected by Ebola at the Gabon-Congo border, appear to be asymptomatically infected.[17] Phylogenetic analysis of viruses isolated from infected people and fruit bats suggests that all genetic variation seen thus far in the Ebola virus type so far studied, including virus amplified from fruit bats, appears to be the product of mutations that have accumulated within the last thirty years. This is a slightly surprising finding, because it seems to contradict the notion of a long association between the virus and its bat reservoir. There are several possible explanations, one of which is that the virus was introduced to these fruit bats around the same time it affected other wildlife populations and emerged in humans. This scenario does not rule out bats as current reservoir species; instead, it would imply that the primary reservoir of the Ebola virus Zaire has yet to be found.[17]

Conclusion

A key step in determining the threat imposed by new pathogens is identifying the route along which they are transmitted from their reservoir to new hosts, such as domestic livestock or humans.[18] In the case of pathogens that use bats as reservoirs, a common route seems likely. Bats fly and so do not ingest large amounts of food. Frequently, the food is chewed and the unwanted residual portion (either fruit remnants or the larger parts of insects) drops to the ground. If the discarded food contains saliva infected with virus particles and is ingested by scavengers—palm civets, primates, domestic animals—a potential pathway to humans develops. Given this scenario, the transmission of emergent pathogens from bats to terrestrial hosts (including people) is unidirectional. Thus, bats transmit SARS coronavirus to palm civets, but not vice versa. This means that control of the disease has to focus on either controlling its abundance in its reservoir, or preventing its spillover between hosts, or rapidly reducing its spread once it has infected humans or domestic livestock.[18] This creates a dilemma for public health and conservation biology. Increased rates of spillover-mediated pathogen transmission from bats to humans or other terrestrial hosts may simply reflect an increase in their contact through anthropogenic modification of the bat's natural environment (the skunk rabies epidemic in Flagstaff provides a good example). It will be difficult to prevent or reduce spillover. On the other hand, we know from our experience of trying to control rabies in terrestrial carnivores that attempts to control potentially emergent pathogens by focusing on their reservoir hosts are also fraught with difficulty.[18]

References

1. C. H. Calisher, J. E. Childs, H. E. Field, K. V. Holmes, and T. Schountz (2006), "Bats: Important Reservoir Hosts of Emerging Viruses," *Clinical Microbiology Reviews* 19: 531–45.

2. S. L. Messenger, C. E. Rupprecht, and J. S. Smith (2003), "Bats, Emerging Virus Infections, and the Rabies Paradigm," in *Bat Ecology*, ed. T. H. Kunz and M. B. Fenton (Chicago: University of Chicago Press), 622–79.

3. S. Vázquez-Morón, A. Avellón, and J. E. Echevarría (2006), "RT-PCR for Detection of All Seven Genotypes of Lyssavirus Genus," *Journal of Virological Methods* 135: 281–87.

4. H. Badrane and N. Tordo (2001), "Host Switching in Lyssavirus History from the Chiroptera to the Carnivora Orders," *Journal of Virology* 75: 8096–101.

5. C. A. Hanlon, I. V. Kuzmin, J. D. Blanton, W. C. Weldon, J. S. Manangan, and C. E. Rupprecht (2005), "Efficacy of Rabies Biologics Against New Lyssaviruses from Eurasia," *Virus Research* 111: 44–54.

6. I. V. Kuzmin, G. J. Hughes, and C. E. Rupprecht (2006), "Phylogenetic Relationships of Seven Previously Unclassified Viruses Within the Family Rhabdoviridae Using Partial Nucleoprotein Gene Sequences," *Journal of General Virology* 87: 2323–31.

7. A. Belotto, L. F. Leanes, M. C. Schneider, H. Tamayo, and E. Correa (2005), "Overview of Rabies in the Americas," *Virus Research* 111: 5–12.

8. G. J. Hughes, L. A. Orciari, and C. E. Rupprecht (2005), "Evolutionary Timescale of Rabies Virus Adaptation to North American Bats Inferred from the Substitution Rate of the Nucleoprotein Gene," *Journal of General Virology* 86: 1467–74.

9. M. J. Leslie, S. Messenger, R. E. Rohde, J. Smith, R. Cheshier, C. Hanlon, and C. E. Rupprecht (2006), "Bat-Associated Rabies Virus in Skunks," *Emerging Infectious Diseases* 12: 1274–77.

10. C. E. Rupprecht, C. A. Hanlon, J. Blanton, J. Manangan, P. Morrill, S. Murphy, M. Niezgoda, L. A. Orciari, C. L. Schumacher, and B. Dietzschold (2005), "Oral Vaccination of Dogs with Recombinant Rabies Virus Vaccines," *Virus Research* 111: 101–5.

11. J. Blancou, M. P. Kieny, R. Lathe, J. P. Lecocq, P. P. Pastore, J. P. Soulebot, and P. Desmettre (1986), "Oral Vaccination of the Fox Against Rabies Using a Live Recombinant Vaccinia Virus," *Nature* 322: 373–75.

12. L.-F. Wang, Z. Shi, S. Zhang, H. Field, P. Daszak, and B. T. Eaton (2006), "Review of Bats and SARS," *Emerging Infectious Diseases* 12: 1834–40.

13. W. Li, Z. Shi, M. Yu, W. Ren, C. Smith, J. H. Epstein, H. Wang, G. Crameri, Z. Hu, H. Zhang, J. Zhang, J. McEachern, H. Field, P. Daszak, B. T. Eaton, S. Zhang, and L.-F. Wang (2005), "Bats Are Natural Reservoirs of SARS-Like Coronaviruses," *Science* 310: 676–79.

14. "Questions and Answers About Ebola Hemorrhagic Fever" (2005), CDC, Special Pathogens Branch, November, http://www.cdc.gov/ncidod/dvrd/Spb/mnpages/dispages/ebola/qa.htm.

15. E. M. Leroy, P. Telfer, B. Kumulungui, P. Yaba, P. Rouquet, P. Roques, J.-P. Gonzalez, T. G. Ksiazek, P. E. Rollin, and E. A. Nerrienet (2004), "Serological Survey of Ebola Virus Infection in Central African Nonhuman Primates," *Journal of Infectious Diseases* 190: 1895–99.

16. E. M. Leroy, B. Kumulungui, X. Pourrut, R. Rouquet, A. Hassanin, P. Yaba, A. Délicat, J. T. Paweska, J.-P. Gonzalez, and R. Swanepoel (2005), "Fruit Bats as Reservoirs of Ebola Virus: Bat Species Eaten by People in Central Africa Show Evidence of Symptomless Ebola Infection," *Nature* 438: 476.

17. R. Biek, P. D. Walsh, E. M. Leroy, and L. A. Real (2006), "Recent Common Ancestry of Ebola Zaire Virus Found in a Bat Reservoir," *PLoS Pathogens* 2: 885–86.

18. A. P. Dobson (2005), "What Links Bats to Emerging Infectious Diseases?" *Science* 310: 628–29.

Part IV
National and Global Responses

Chapter 14
International Efforts at Detection and Control

François-Xavier Meslin and Corrie Brown

Emerging zoonotic diseases are increasingly recognized as a global and regional issue with potentially serious human health and economic impacts. Over the past decades, viruses and other agents causing many previously unknown human infectious diseases emerged from animal reservoirs. Some examples are human immunodeficiency virus (HIV), Ebola virus, West Nile virus, Nipah virus, Hantavirus, and more recently the agent causing sudden acute respiratory syndrome (SARS) and the H5N1 strain of highly pathogenic avian influenza (HPAI) virus. In 2004, the World Health Organization (WHO), the UN Food and Agriculture Organization (FAO), and the World Organisation for Animal Health (OIE) adopted a common definition: "an emerging zoonosis is a zoonosis that is newly recognized or newly evolved, or that has occurred previously but shows an increase in incidence or expansion in geographical, host or vector range." Many zoonoses that are endemic but epidemic-prone, such as leptospirosis, brucellosis, and rabies, would therefore also fit the definition. In addition, as demonstrated by HPAI in birds, emerging diseases of yesterday quickly become endemic diseases of today.

History shows that the cascade of events leading to the emergence of a new disease is different each time; nevertheless, several processes are known to favor such emergence. These include microbiological adaptation, environmental changes, the globalization of agriculture, food production, and trade, and human behavioral factors. Predicting which zoonotic diseases may arise in the future is extremely difficult, however, owing to the multifactorial and evolving nature of the risk factors involved (although vector-transmitted infections may prove an exception because they are strongly influenced by environmental factors). Even so, the effective prevention or rapid containment of future emergence events will require the early and accurate detection of new outbreaks of epidemic diseases (including emerging zoonoses), an improved capacity for understanding the underlying causes of disease emergence, and a better understanding of the ecology of the agents and their hosts.

International Organizations and Early Warning Systems

There are three key international organizations involved in global surveillance for emerging infectious diseases. The OIE consists of 169 member countries. One of the objectives of the OIE is to promote transparency, and this function is evident at the annual general meeting, when the chief veterinary officers of the 167 countries get together to discuss international issues. The OIE acts to harmonize relevant trade requirements and strives to help member countries, especially developing countries, improve their veterinary services and overall infrastructure. In return, member countries have certain responsibilities; for example, they must report the occurrence of up to 130 listed diseases (although the only real penalty for failure to report is losing credibility with other member countries). The FAO helps developing nations deal with transboundary animal diseases (in the United States these are called foreign animal diseases, or FADs) and manages an emergency prevention system (EMPRES). The rinderpest program is the FAO's biggest program, but it also works on a whole alphabet soup of diseases: pleuropneumonia, foot-and-mouth disease, peste des petits ruminants, Newcastle disease, lumpy skin disease, African swine fever, and avian influenza. Several developing countries have FAO laboratories, which are often the only functioning facilities in the country. In 2006, in collaboration with the OIE, the FAO established a Crisis Management Center in Rome (with funding from the U. S. Department of Agriculture, France, Germany, Italy, the Netherlands, and the UK). The purpose of the center is to help control and contain dangerous diseases, including H5N1 HPAI. Like the OIE, WHO requires that its member countries report certain diseases, and like the OIE it works to improve transparency. For example, in 2000 WHO established the Global Outbreak Alert Response Network (GOARN), a network that included not just the official members of WHO but many affiliates (such as the Red Cross, the Red Crescent, and Médecins Sans Frontières), which were brought together to help in information gathering and preparedness planning.

In 2004, the OIE, FAO, and WHO jointly reported their intent to integrate the early warning, alert, and response systems each organization had developed independently to facilitate early detection of potentially linked animal and public health events. This new initiative was called the Global Early Warning System for Transboundary Animal Diseases (GLEWS). GLEWS represents a valuable platform for enhancing global early warning and response to zoonotic disease outbreaks. GLEWS is meant to promote detection, transparency, preparedness, and integrated surveillance. Each organization brings something different to GLEWS. The OIE is involved in efforts to improve transparency. Governments have all kinds of economic and political reasons for not reporting disease, so the role of the OIE is to try and persuade ministries of agriculture to report diseases more consistently. It will also help with developing animal health infrastructure. The FAO, on the other hand, contributes its emergency management expertise (for example, EMPRES). WHO, which has a very strong track record in monitoring diseases and mounting responses, offers a much better communications network than either the OIE or the FAO.

While international integration at this level is an important step toward the creation of an effective early warning system for emerging disease, we should also seek new mechanisms for early warning, surveillance, and response. This would also require using new approaches (such as syndromic surveillance) and new tools (such as mathematical modeling, geographic information systems, and satellite remote sensing), which should be used in combination for best effect. The study of the transmission dynamics and control of infectious diseases is increasingly based on mathematical or computational models. Mathematical models are formulated and analyzed to achieve a better understanding of observed patterns (for example, the key determinants of a disease pattern) and how different interventions introduced at different times after the emergence of an epidemic might influence the future incidence of infection and associated disease. Successful modeling efforts involve integrating the tools and approaches of different disciplines, including medical, veterinary, and population biology; research; field monitoring and reporting of wildlife health issues; information technology; economics; the social sciences; and diagnostics. Satellite remote sensing of land surface conditions and atmospheric dynamics can provide important information relevant to understanding the coupling between and among climate variability, ecological dynamics, and zoonotic disease outbreak patterns, and satellite remote sensing products from a variety of platforms can provide information on cloud cover, rainfall, temperature, and vegetation conditions that are relevant to the emergence, propagation, and abundance of vectors that transmit various zoonotic diseases.

Advanced surveillance systems exist in a few countries, but most countries, especially developing countries, are ill-equipped to develop, implement, and maintain such systems. Emerging zoonotic diseases are likely to occur in countries that have the weakest infrastructures for detection and response. In light of recent global events, such as the emergence of SARS and HPAI, there is an urgent need to enhance the capacity of these countries, and subsequently to connect the various surveillance and early warning, alert, and response systems at the regional and international levels.

The new (2005) International Health Regulations are an international legal instrument whose purpose and scope are to prevent or control the international spread of disease by providing an appropriate public health response. Under the new regulations, emphasis must be placed on building the appropriate preparedness and response capacity in countries and linking the capacity to regional and international networks.

New Approaches for Responding to Emerging Zoonotic Outbreaks

A biphasic approach should be considered for handling emerging zoonoses: a short- to intermediate-term response to an outbreak or emergence event, indicated by an increasing number of cases (in either animals or humans), and a long-term comprehensive study of the ecology of the zoonotic pathogen. The short-term response should include setting up two emergency teams to respond quickly to the disease outbreak or emergence event. The first team should primarily be responsible for infection control by creating a case definition, identifying the mechanism of disease transmission, and breaking the chain of transmission, thus preventing new cases. The second team should concurrently undertake studies on the disease ecology by compiling current knowledge about the disease and using this knowledge to conduct preliminary animal surveys to identify the etiological agent. The two teams would be responsible for implementing short-term control measures and should determine whether or not there is a need for long-term follow-up studies by assessing the likelihood of recurrence or emergence in new areas.

A number of control methods and tools currently available at the animal reservoir, vector, and human levels would be appropriate for the prevention and control of emerging zoonotic diseases. For domestic animals, the common methods and tools used in disease control are vaccination of pets or livestock (such as vaccination for rabies control), the prophylactic use of antiparasitics (such as antitrypanosomals or coccidiostats), proper biosecurity and quarantine measures (such as excluding wildlife from domestic stock and mandating hygienic practices in husbandry and among farm workers), eradication programs (depopulation), appropriate veterinary care, and comprehensive herd health programs (for example, breeding for disease resistance, feed and water control, using best animal husbandry practices, practicing routine disease surveillance, and testing animals before they enter or leave a farm). Disease surveillance and control in wild animals should take into consideration a number of conservation issues, particularly the conservation status of the species under investigation. The following methods and tools may be used after careful evaluation of the species involved and its ecology: isolation and the creation of physical barriers to exclude wild animals from farms or human residences, population control by culling, treating, and vaccinating defined populations (an example is the oral rabies vaccination of foxes), limiting wildlife movement, conducting preliminary testing of all live import and exports, and exercising care in adopting and translocating wild animals.

Vector control is an effective tool in the prevention and control of vector-borne zoonotic diseases, for example by spraying against fleas and mosquitoes during plague and Rift Valley fever outbreaks, respectively, and using tick control in outbreaks of Crimean Congo hemorrhagic fever and Lyme disease. Other effective methods involve environmental management through elimination of vector breeding habitats, as well as limiting anthropogenic activities that promote vector breeding, such as land clearing, unplanned development, and the destruction of habitats that support vector predators.

Strengthening National, Regional, and International Capacities for Zoonotic Surveillance, Prevention, and Control

As the emergence of a disease in any given place on the planet may ultimately have consequences for everybody, resource-rich countries should invest in the establishment and strengthening of surveillance systems in resource-limited countries as an acknowledgment of the international significance of emerging zoonoses. To facilitate the much-needed international and national capacity strengthening for zoonotic surveillance, prevention, and control (or elimination), international organizations such as WHO, the FAO, and the OIE should promote the value of surveillance to their member countries.

A great deal of knowledge and information relevant to the detection of emerging zoonotic events of public health significance already exists in many countries. Each member country should establish a system to obtain, collate, and analyze relevant data centrally. The international organizations should also ensure full implementation of the joint GLEWS agreement signed by WHO, the FAO, and the OIE to allow the detection of potentially linked animal and public health events. They should also encourage research to investigate the usefulness of surveillance data from novel systems (vector population monitoring, meteorological data, land surface scanning, animal and human demographics) for advance warning of zoonotic public health events. Where applicable, such systems should be implemented at a national level (an example here is the early warning systems for Rift Valley fever based on climatic data). These early warning and response systems should be organized so that they can rapidly incorporate the results of research into novel surveillance methods, and they should provide a mechanism for gathering data and information from satellite remote sensing platforms that can be analyzed quickly so that the system provides close to real-time monitoring of conditions associated with zoonotic disease outbreaks. It is a responsibility of the international organizations to encourage research on new approaches to the transport of laboratory specimens (such as the transport of inactivated samples containing DNA and RNA) and handling pathogens; to facilitate analysis of the biodiversity of potential pathogens in animal populations (such as the Lyssaviruses; see Chapter 13); to support the upstream detection of agents of potential zoonotic significance; to fund research leading to the development and use of inexpensive, sensitive, and specific rapid diagnostic tests for field situations; and to elicit political awareness of and support for the implementation of a public and animal health infrastructure to address zoonotic disease issues. Individual countries should establish sustained personnel interchange between ministries of agriculture and ministries of health. If veterinary and public health personnel become familiar with each other before a crisis, they will be better positioned to resolve the inevitable differences that arise during an animal or human health emergency. Countries should also integrate animal and human health data at a national level, implement systems for the identification and localization of commercial animal herds or flocks and for tracking national and international livestock movements, and conduct cost-benefit assessments to demonstrate the benefits of such practices in the prevention and control of zoonotic disease. In each country, there should be an intersectoral committee for zoonoses preparedness and control (to create, for example, national preparedness plans for an outbreak response). Such committees should include representatives of relevant public and animal health agencies and national reference laboratories. This multisector approach should also extend to networks that are designed to detect and respond to emerging zoonotic infections and to monitor changes in known or potential risk factors for the emergence of zoonotic disease. These networks should include nontraditional partners, such as nongovernmental organizations (for example, wildlife organizations) and zoos. The consequences of changes in policy or common practice should also be carefully considered. Countries should consider the negative impact on the environment, endemic wildlife species, and the public health of national projects that promote mixed animal farming (say) or the introduction of large-scale, single-species animal production systems or disease control programs. Such assessments should examine the risk of new zoonotic agents emerging as a result of the change in practice or policy.

Conclusion

The creation of a global early warning system for emerging diseases by integrating the existing expertise of international organizations such as the OIE, the FAO, and WHO is an important step, but we must continue to investigate novel approaches to detection and response. To this end, nontraditional stakeholders (nongovernmental organizations) must be involved at all levels of the process.[1]

Reference

1. World Health Organization (2004), Report of the WHO/FAO/OIE Joint Consultation on Emerging Zoonotic Diseases, organized in collaboration with the Health Council of the Netherlands, Geneva, May 3–5, whqlibdoc.who.int/hq/2004/WHO_CDS_CPE_ZFK_2004.9.pdf.

Chapter 15
The Public Health Workforce

Hugh Mainzer

An emergency public health response usually reflects either missed opportunities to plan and practice good prevention or an inadequate understanding of the vulnerabilities in a population or in a public health system. For example, approximately one-quarter of the global disease burden and more than one-third of the disease burden among children is due to modifiable environmental factors. An estimated 94 percent of diarrheal cases are associated with risk factors such as unsafe drinking water, poor sanitation, and hygiene.[1] The majority of health care spending is directed toward medical care and biomedical research. However, behavior and the environment are responsible for more than 70 percent of avoidable deaths.[2] Since few of the chapters in this book have focused on environmental issues per se (but see Chapter 6), this chapter attempts to redress the balance and define the activities that might constitute veterinary public health in the widest possible context. A recent World Health Organization Technical Report defined veterinary public health as "the sum of all contributions to the physical, mental, and social well-being of humans through an understanding and application of veterinary science."[3] This chapter proceeds in that spirit.

Veterinarians and the Public Health Workforce

Veterinarians are part of a much bigger team of public health professionals who are practicing public health. In fact, veterinarians are estimated to make up less than 1 percent of the public health workforce.[4] However, because veterinarians work at the interface of human, animal, and environmental health, they are uniquely positioned to view health through the lens of public health impact.[5] Veterinarians can and should be part of all the whole range of public health activities, but the profession tends to limit itself to diagnostics, disease monitoring, enforcement of disease control policies, and research. The profession should be involved in all the activities that make up public health. It is in the veterinary oath, taken on completion of clinical training: "I solemnly swear to use my scientific knowledge and skills for the benefit of society through the protection of animal health, the relief of animal suffering, the conservation of animal resources, the promotion of public health and the advancement of medical knowledge."[6] Veterinarians should break out of the traditional realms of food safety and zoonoses.

What should be the role of the public health veterinarian in the modern era? It certainly includes policy making, public health program management and leadership, and the application of epidemiology and risk assessment methodology. It should also include acquiring and acting on expertise in laboratory animal, herd health and population health issues, food safety, food animal disease control, zoonosis prevention and control, and disease prevention and control globally. Veterinarians should be prepared to work with environmental health specialists—sanitary engineers, industrial hygienists, those professionals formerly known as sanitarians—and become familiar with a systems approach to public health. Veterinarians are turning to environmental health scientists and practitioners to develop their understanding that many outbreaks and public health emergencies are failures of veterinary prevention infrastructure. It has been demonstrated that the professions can work together to investigate the environmental antecedents that lead to adverse health outcomes.[5,7]

Changing Approaches to Disease Outbreak Investigation and Control

In the United States, veterinarians interested in the interface of human and animal health often become Epidemic Intelligence Service (EIS) officers with the Centers for Disease Control and Prevention. When EIS officers conduct outbreak investigations, they seek (among other things) to identify those measures that would have prevented or facilitated faster intervention. Unfortunately, in the past, when those system modifications were put in place after the response had wound down, the officers did not always measure the effectiveness of the suggested modifications. Veterinarians need to broaden their view of what tasks constitute the practice of public health. They need to respond to the impacted health or safety system in its totality. Another example from the food industry is relevant here. Traditionally, EIS officers looked for the smoking gun: they looked for the sick food handler, the cross-connected pipe, or the bad tuna or raspberry or spinach. More recently, though, they have begun looking analytically at all the processes—equipment, people, and economics—that influence food safety. In the past, sick food handlers were often fired, creating a strong disincentive to report illness. To overcome that problem, public health professionals, including veterinarians, are working with the retail food industry in several states to teach food managers how to evaluate and train food harvesters, handlers, and preparers and how not to disincentivize reporting illness. Similarly, the food-borne disease outbreak in the United States attributed to *Escherichia coli* contamination of spinach prompted a disease investigation that included environmentalists and engineers working with state health and agriculture authorities (and FDA officials) to examine all the inputs that led to this contamination. It was important to know that spinach was the vehicle, but it was also important to know all the factors and processes that led to the outbreak.

Veterinary Public Health Issues That Do Not Involve Infectious Disease

What are the response priorities following a natural disaster such as a hurricane? Infectious disease control usually comes to mind as the having the highest response priority, but the true number one priority after a natural disaster is providing water to affected populations. Access to food, shelter, basic sanitation, hazard assessment and disease/injury surveillance, and basic health-care services is also essential for both humans and animals affected by the calamity. In the United States especially, veterinarians will increasingly be involved in response and recover operations following natural disasters. After Hurricane Katrina, President Bush signed a new law that requires states' emergency management agencies and mass sheltering facilities to provide shelter for pet animals locally or regionally in the case of a disaster, act of terror, or public health emergency. Each state, as part of its emergency preparedness plan, must create a shelter plan that provides for pets as well as people. State authorities are turning to veterinarians, especially those with public health and preventive medicine training and experience, to craft animal shelter plans. The role of public health practitioners in emergencies is to assist the community and its population when resources are overwhelmed or nonexistent. Organized public health often has to support and augment the infrastructure and the whole range of public health disease and disability prevention programs throughout prolonged community recovery and rebuilding activities. Veterinarians have the skills and the education to be able to assist in that effort and do the job well.

What Do Public Health Veterinarians Do?

Public health veterinarians are public health policy makers; public health or environmental health program managers and executives, epidemiologists; community practitioners; local, state, federal, or international health officers; public health laboratory scientists; public health educators and communications experts; animal control consultants and shelter medicine practitioners; occupational safety and health advisers; and teachers of public health sciences and preventive medicine. They are also subject matter experts on zoonoses, vector-borne disease, and even noninfectious disease prevention and control programs. Typical activities involve environmental risk assessment and the study of health hazard effects; ecological and environmental health sciences; disease surveillance; conservation medicine practice; quarantine services and select agent oversight; maintenance of food and water safety; biomedical research; drug and medical device quality and safety assurance; agricultural program, nutritional guideline, and sustainable community development consultation; food animal disease control activities; global health improvement programs (including malaria control and HIV/AIDS prevention); biological, chemical, and radiologic terrorism preparedness, prevention, and response; and natural and technological disaster and pandemic preparedness, prevention, and response.[5]

A 2002 survey of veterinary schools in the United States came to the following conclusions: "Veterinary students are exposed to a median of sixty hours of public health, epidemiology, and preventive medicine in required stand-alone courses in these areas. Four veterinary schools also have required rotations for senior students in public health, preventive medicine, or population medicine. Contact time for required public health, epidemiology, and preventive medicine courses ranges from 30 to 150 contact hours. Advanced training was available in these subjects at 79 percent of the twenty-seven schools."[8] Nevertheless, in the United States, there are just under three times as many public health physicians as there are public health veterinarians. Although there are not a lot more physicians than veterinarians in public health, physicians have much more influence in the leadership of population health programs and initiatives. Veterinarians could and should assume a larger role. The veterinary profession could and should integrate the practice of veterinary medicine closely with the mainstream practice of public health by recruiting into veterinary schools more faculty members, as well as students, who are looking for clinical training and who already have knowledge, technical skills, or experience in population health or preventive medicine. To improve the veterinary profession's participation in global public health practice, the analytic skill sets, herd/population health problem-solving methodologies, and clinical foundations so necessary for the protection and improvement of human as well as animal well-being should be promoted, taught, and financed in veterinary schools and veterinary professional organizations across the globe.

The author's views do not necessarily represent the official policy or programs of the U.S. Centers for Disease Control and Prevention or the U.S. Department of Health and Human Services.

References

1. A. Prüss-Üstün and C. Corvalán (2006), Preventing Disease Through Healthy Environments: Towards an Estimate of the Environmental Burden of Disease, WHO Report, http://www.who.int/quantifying_ehimpacts/publications/preventingdisease/en/index.html.

2. Institute of Medicine (2002), The Future of the Public's Health in the 21st Century, http://books.nap.edu/catalog.php?record_id=10548.

3. World Health Organization (2002), Future Trends in Veterinary Public Health: Report of a WHO Study Group, WHO Technical Report Series No. 907, http://libdoc.who.int/trs/WHO_TRS_907.pdf.

4. K. Gebbie (2000), The Public Health Workforce Enumeration 2000 (New York: Center for Health Policy, Columbia School of Nursing).

5. H. Mainzer (2006), "Veterinarians and Environmental Health Practitioners: Partners in Prevention," Journal of Environmental Health 69: 60–61.

6. American Veterinary Medical Association (1999), Veterinarian's Oath, http://www.avma.org/about_avma/whoweare/oath.asp.

7. J. Cassady, C. Higgins, H. Mainzer, S. Seys, J. Sarisky, and K. Musgrave (2006), "Beyond Compliance: Environmental Health Problem Solving, Interagency Collaboration, and Risk Assessment to Prevent Waterborne Disease Outbreaks," Journal of Epidemiology and Community Health 60: 672–74.

8. C. Riddle, H. Mainzer, and M. Julian (2003), "Training the Veterinary Public Health Workforce: A Review of Educational Opportunities in United States Veterinary Schools," Journal of Veterinary Medical Education 31: 161–67.

Chapter 16
The Task Ahead

Alan M. Kelly

This book focuses our attention on the difficult global challenges facing the veterinary profession in the twenty-first century. It lays out the case for a global strategy, incorporating the profession's traditional responsibilities in a new paradigm aimed at protecting and preserving our planet's resources so that humans and nature can coexist without irreparable damage to Earth's biodiversity and ecological integrity. Veterinary schools in particular face an immediate challenge in determining how best to educate more students in public and ecosystem health. Because these are political as well as medical issues, students need exposure to the political and economic issues surrounding globalization.

At a World Health Organization conference in 1999, veterinary public health was defined as "the sum of all contributions to the physical, mental and social well-being of humans through an understanding and application of veterinary science." A definition this broad encompasses virtually every aspect of the profession's functions in serving society. While the traditional elements of food safety, disease surveillance, and prevention remain central concerns, a global dimension adds new levels of complexity, with special emphasis on strategies for the alleviation of world hunger, environmental preservation, including biodiversity of animal species, and responses to acts of bioterrorism. Such a broad spectrum of responsibilities blurs the distinctions between and among food animal medicine, wildlife medicine, microbiology, epidemiology, and public and ecosystem health. To succeed, the profession must also address the political aspects of its broadened mission, communicating forcefully the need for investment in rural farming economies and for advancing the efficiency and profitability of multinational livestock and poultry operations that flourish in the global marketplace.

The Challenge

If present projections hold, the world's population will increase 50 percent by 2050. During the same period, driven by urbanization and the emergence of a middle class in developing nations, the demand for foods of animal origin is expected to treble. For rich and poor countries alike, the resulting growth in trade will increase the risk of contamination of foodstuffs with infectious agents. As a consequence, the need for veterinary intervention to control disease outbreaks in poultry, livestock, and fish will grow proportionately.

Many of the infectious agents that have emerged in the past two decades originated in wildlife reservoirs. As people intrude more and more on wildlife habitats, and as the sale of bushmeat continues to flourish, more outbreaks can be expected to follow. While disease outbreaks, which often appear without warning, are most prevalent in and cause greatest damage to developing countries, developed nations in a globalized economy are also at risk. In Chapter 14, François-Xavier Meslin and Corrie Brown described how several government and nongovernmental agencies are responding to the challenge. The question for veterinary schools is how to design and implement curricula and how to attract more students to meet the present and future need for more veterinarians trained in veterinary public and ecosystem health. Risk assessment and management, mathematical modeling of disease patterns and distribution, and the impact of environmental factors such as global warming will require greater emphasis than students now receive in veterinary public health offerings. Some exposure to political science and anthropology is also needed if graduates are to participate more effectively in developing international policies on disease control and public health. These are crucial challenges, for multinational corporations, driven by the need to capture markets and make profits, dominate trade in livestock and poultry, with little concern for ecosystem health or the survival of millions of small rural farmers, who find themselves increasingly detached from the global economy.

To meet the rising demand for animal protein, many developing countries are seeing an expansion in the numbers of livestock- and poultry-intensive production units. In addition to economies of scale, advantages include improved production efficiency and disease control. Large concentrations of animals, however, bring their own set of controversial issues, among them animal welfare concerns and opportunities for the emergence of novel or multidrug-resistant pathogens. These issues, highly relevant to global veterinary public health and food animal veterinary practice in general, should inform veterinary school curricular reform and development. Instruction in animal health management and economics, nutrition, reproduction, and biosecurity is essential to prepare students for managerial positions in intensive production animal agriculture.

Intensive livestock and poultry operations are commonly located near cities in the developing world, where they benefit from the generally good local infrastructure, an abundant and accessible energy supply, and, often, an absence of environmental regulations or enforcement. Typically, inexpensive waste disposal methods result in air and water pollution and in the dissemination of waterborne diseases. The Americanization of markets in Southeast Asia is evident in the degree of integration of intensive livestock operations with supermarkets and fast food chains. In addition to squeezing out small farmers, large animal production operations in peri-urban areas are not sustainable. Animal waste cannot continue to be dumped into streams and rivers that are already wretchedly polluted; the incidence of algal blooms is rising and fisheries are in decline. To avoid impending catastrophe, developing countries must invest in transportation systems that will allow intensive livestock and poultry operations to relocate to areas where land is available and waste disposal can be managed responsibly. Investment in better rural transportation systems would bring additional returns by helping rural farmers, with their small, vulnerable, mixed livestock operations, to survive. The migration of young people to the cities, the loss of local markets, and lack of access to global markets have marginalized millions of small farmers. Owing to hot, humid conditions, poor infrastructure, and distant urban markets, many smallholders face losses of up to 30 percent of their post-harvest produce. Serving the needs of small farmers is among the veterinary profession's most difficult global challenges.

A Different Focus

The medical profession's focus on tuberculosis, malaria, and especially the HIV/AIDS epidemic has diverted resources from efforts to build a comprehensive public health infrastructure. Inadvertently, this narrow focus has magnified the challenges facing the veterinary profession at a time when pastoral farming and live animal markets are the most common sources of zoonotic and epizoonotic diseases, the control of which requires a well-integrated veterinary-medical public health infrastructure. Finding the resources to accomplish this goal will require determined leadership and the long-term involvement of veterinarians at the very highest levels of policy development. Moreover, veterinary schools, in order to attract and train larger numbers of veterinarians in public and ecosystem health, will require substantially greater investment by governmental and nongovernmental agencies than is presently the case.

Contributors

D. J. Alexander, O.B.E., worked at Veterinary Laboratories Agency in Weybridge, UK, for more than thirty years. Now retired from the VLA, he continues to work as a poultry and virology consultant for international organizations and governmental bodies, including the EU. In 2002 he was awarded the Robert Fraser Gordon Memorial Medal for distinguished contributions to poultry science, and in 2006 he received the World Organisation for Animal Health meritorious award, the Médaille du Mérite.

Gregg W. BeVier is CEO of AgGlobalVision, one of the world's leading animal health companies. His background includes livestock genetics, animal health, and integrated livestock production operations. He holds a D.V.M. and an M.B.A. from the University of Illinois and has authored a number of articles in journals and proceedings and co-authored several book chapters, all related to swine reproductive physiology. BeVier is a lifetime member of the American Veterinary Medicine Association and the American Association of Swine Veterinarians and serves on the Dean's Advisory Council at the College of Veterinary Medicine, University of Illinois.

Corrie Brown is Professor and Head of the Department of Veterinary Pathology at the University of Georgia College of Veterinary Medicine. She also serves as coordinator of International Veterinary Medicine for the College of Veterinary Medicine at the University of Georgia.

Ilaria Capua heads the Virology Department at the Istituto Zooprofilattico Sperimentale delle Venezie in Italy and also directs the Food and Agriculture Organization and World Organisation for Animal Health reference laboratories for avian influenza and Newcastle disease. In 2000 she developed the DIVA (Differentiating Vaccinated from Infected Animals) strategy, based on heterologous vaccination, to combat avian influenza.

Darin S. Carroll is employed by the Centers for Disease Control in the Division of Viral and Rickettsial Diseases Poxvirus program. He has participated in disease outbreak and surveillance investigations of arenaviruses, Hantaviruses, Ebola, monkeypox, and Nipah virus. His research emphasis is on increasing the knowledge of the ecology and evolution of viral zoonoses and their associated hosts in order to better predict outbreaks and identify ways to decrease human exposure risks.

Bruno B. Chomel joined the faculty of the School of Veterinary Medicine at the University of California, Davis, in 1990, where he is Professor of Zoonoses. His research centers on cat scratch disease and *Bartonella* infections in domestic animals and wildlife, the epidemiology of rabies and plague, and the zoonoses of wildlife. He has been Director of the World Health Organization/Pan American Health Organization Collaborating Center on New and Emerging Zoonoses since 1997, and was Director of the Master of Preventive Veterinary Medicine at the University of California, Davis, from 1998 until 2001.

David T. Galligan is Professor of Animal Health Economics at the University of Pennsylvania School of Veterinary Medicine. His area of academic interest is the economic cost of animal diseases, as well as management and production inefficiency in modern animal production systems. His current research is in how farm management decision making influences the cost of animal disease through the use of real options analysis.

Cornelis (Cees) de Haan was from 1992 until his retirement in 2001 the senior adviser for livestock development at the World Bank, where he was responsible for the bank's livestock development policies. He remains a consultant on animal agriculture for the bank. He previously served as a senior scientist and Deputy Director General for Research at the International Livestock Center for Africa in Addis Ababa. De Haan joined the World Bank in Washington, D.C., in 1983, initially as senior livestock specialist for West Africa and later for Eastern Europe and the Middle East.

David Harlan is Director of Global Animal Health and Food Safety at Cargill, an international provider of food, agricultural, and risk management products and services with 149,000 employees in sixty-three countries. He joined Cargill in 2002 when it acquired Taylor Packing Company, where he was Assistant Vice President of Marketing and Technical Affairs.

Joan Hendricks graduated with a B.S. in biology and psychology from Yale University. In 1979 and 1980 she was awarded a V.M.D. and a Ph.D. from the School of Veterinary Medicine at the University of Pennsylvania, where she remained to complete a residency and postdoctoral fellowship. She is the twelfth Dean of the School of Veterinary Medicine at the University of Pennsylvania and the third female dean of a veterinary school in the United States. Hendricks served on the faculty of the school for more than twenty years. In 2001 she was named Henry and Corinne R. Bower Professor of Small Animal Medicine, becoming the first woman to hold an endowed professorship at the school. In addition to serving as Chief of Critical Care in the Department of Clinical Studies (Philadelphia), she is Founding Director of the Veterinary Clinical Investigation Center and holds a secondary appointment as Professor in the Department of Medicine at Penn's School of Medicine.

Candace Jacobs is Vice President of Quality Assurance and Environmental Affairs at H-E-B Foods. She is responsible for food safety and sanitation at more than 300 stores in Texas and northern Mexico and also oversees the company's brand quality assurance program, product quality laboratory, and environmental compliance. From 2000 to 2005 she was Director of Scientific and Regulatory Affairs at the Coca-Cola Company, in which capacity she was responsible for all aspects of North America product compliance with FDA food regulations, as well as global company scientific and regulatory initiatives, activities, reporting, and partnerships.

Edward Kanara is Senior Director of Strategic Initiatives for Veterinary Medicine Research and Development at Pfizer Animal Health. Since joining Pfizer in 1990, he has led various teams, including Veterinary Operations, Drug Safety and Pharmacovigilance, Vaccine Discovery Research, and most recently Infectious Disease, Immunotherapy, and Oncology Discovery Research.

Alan M. Kelly completed his undergraduate work at the University of Reading and received his veterinary degree from the University of Bristol, both in the UK. He came to the University of Pennsylvania in 1962, within a month of graduating, on a National Cancer Institute fellowship and received his doctorate in pathology from Penn in 1967. He joined the faculty of the School of Veterinary Medicine the following year. Dean Kelly served as chair of the school's Department of Pathobiology from 1990 until 1994. He stepped down as the Gilbert S. Kahn Dean of the School of Veterinary Medicine in 2005 after nearly twelve years, including a first year as Interim Dean. His research interests include muscle disease and muscular dystrophy. Kelly is a member of the Royal College of Veterinary Surgeons, the American Society for Cell Biology, and the Pennsylvania Muscle Institute. He received the university's Lindback Award for Distinguished Teaching in 1974.

Stephen J. Kobrin is William H. Wurster Professor of Multinational Management at the Wharton School, the University of Pennsylvania. His research interests include globalization, global governance, global strategy, and the politics of international business. He is a Fellow of the World Economic Forum and was a rapporteur for the 2003 annual meeting.

Richard Langan, an affiliate Associate Professor of Zoology at the University of New Hampshire, is Director of the university's Atlantic Marine Aquaculture Center and the center's Open Ocean Aquaculture Project, which develops environmentally sound practices and advanced technology for raising native cold-water finfish and shellfish in exposed oceanic environments. He is also Codirector of the NOAA-UNH Cooperative Institute for Coastal and Estuarine Environmental Technology, which develops tools and technologies for clean water and healthy coastal habitats nationwide. He previously worked as a commercial fisherman and owner and operator of seafood and shellfish aquaculture businesses.

Hugh Mainzer joined the CDC's National Center for Environmental Health in 2001 as a senior preventive medicine officer and supervisory epidemiologist in the U.S. Public Health Service with the rank of captain. He is currently assigned to the CDC at the National Center for Environmental Health in its Division of Emergency and Environmental Health Services. He is also a Clinical Assistant Professor in the Department of Environmental and Population Health at the Cummings School of Veterinary Medicine at Tufts University and an Adjunct Instructor in the Department of Community Medicine and Family Health at Tufts University School of Medicine.

François-Xavier Meslin is manager for the World Health Organization of an intercountry project for human and dog rabies prevention and control and also provides oversight of the WHO Zoonoses Control Program in the Mediterranean area. He has worked in Thailand on livestock development and in West Africa on an animal production and health project.

Shelley Rankin is Assistant Professor and Clinician Educator of Microbiology at the Matthew J. Ryan Veterinary Hospital of the University of Pennsylvania and Chief of the Clinical Microbiology Service at Penn. Her primary research focus has been the molecular epidemiology and surveillance of novel strains of *Salmonella* and other enteric pathogens from veterinary and human sources as a control measure in the prevention of disease outbreaks.

Leslie A. Real joined the Emory University faculty in 1998 as Asa Griggs Candler Professor of Biology. He is Director of the Emory Center for Disease Ecology, a multischool initiative exploring the ecological and evolutionary conditions for infectious disease emergence and spread. He is also Director of the Graduate Program in Population Biology, Ecology, and Evolution. His research focuses on the ecology and evolution of infectious diseases and the molecular evolution of viral pathogenesis.

Bruce A. Rideout is a pathologist and disease investigation specialist for the Zoological Society of San Diego (San Diego Zoo and San Diego Wild Animal Park). He joined the Zoological Society in 1991 and is now Head of the Wildlife Disease Laboratories and Associate Director of Conservation and Research for Endangered Species. He is also a research fellow of the Peregrine Fund and an adjunct faculty member at San Diego State University. His primary interests include pathogenesis and epidemiology of infectious diseases, avian embryonic and neonatal pathology as it relates to captive propagation for recovery programs, population dynamics of infectious disease, and disease risk assessment for translocation and reintroduction programs.

Charles Rupprecht is Chief of the Rabies Section, Viral and Rickettsial Zoonoses branch, Division of Viral and Rickettsial Diseases, National Center for Infectious Disease, Centers for Disease Control and Prevention. He is also Director of the World Health Organization Collaborating Center for Rabies Reference and Research, Centers for Disease Control and Prevention, Atlanta, and Adjunct Professor, Population Biology, Ecology, and Evolution Training Program, Emory University.

Gary Smith is Professor of Population Biology and Epidemiology at the School of Veterinary Medicine at the University of Pennsylvania. He has been Chief of the Section of Epidemiology and Public Health since 1995. He has a secondary appointment in the Department of Biostatistics and Epidemiology at Penn's School of Medicine and is an Associate Scholar in the Center for Clinical Epidemiology and Biostatistics, as well as an affiliated faculty member of Penn's Institute for Strategic Threat Analysis and Response and a faculty associate of the Penn Institute of Urban Studies. Currently a standing member of the Microbiology and Infectious Disease Review Committee for the National Institutes of Health, he has been a specialist editor for more than half a dozen scientific journals and now serves as on the editorial review board for the *International Journal of Applied Research in Veterinary Medicine*. His research deals with the epidemiology and population dynamics of infectious diseasees in humans and in wild and domestic animal species.

Lord Soulsby of Swaffham Prior is a distinguished microbiologist and parasitologist. He was created a Life Peer in 1990 as Baron Soulsby of Swaffham Prior, in the County of Cambridgeshire, and sits as a Conservative peer in the House of Lords. Lord Soulsby was a Veterinary Officer for the City of Edinburgh from 1949 to 1952, and then a lecturer in Clinical Parasitology at the University of Bristol from 1952 to 1954. From 1954 to 1963 he was a lecturer in Animal Pathology at the University of Cambridge. He served as Professor of Parasitology at the University of Pennsylvania until 1978, when he returned to the University of Cambridge as Professor of Animal Pathology. He is an honorary member of numerous international parasitology societies and has received several honorary degrees and awards. He has been a Fellow of Wolfson College Cambridge since 1978. Lord Soulsby has been a member of the Council of the Royal College of Veterinary Surgeons since 1978 and is a past President of the Royal Society of Medicine, past President of the Royal College of Veterinary Surgeons, and Emeritus Fellow of Wolfson College, Cambridge. He is President of the Parliamentary and Scientific Committee and President of the Royal Institute of Public Health, and also veterinary surgeon to Her Majesty Queen Elizabeth II. He has published fourteen books as well as articles in various veterinary journals.

Henning P. Steinfeld is Head of the Livestock Sector Analysis and Policy Branch at the Food and Agriculture Organization in Rome. He has been working on livestock policy for the last fifteen years, focusing on environmental issues, poverty alleviation, and public health protection. He previously worked in agricultural development project in a number of African countries.

Paul B. Thompson is W. K. Kellogg Professor of Philosophy and Agriculture Economics at Michigan State University. He has written extensively on ethical and environmental issues in contemporary agriculture. His book *The Spirit of the Soil: Agriculture and Environmental Ethics* (1995) was one of the first philosophical discussions of farming, and *Sacred Cows and Hot Potatoes: Agrarian Myths and Policy Realities* (1992, with four co-authors) won the American Agricultural Economics Association Award for Excellence in Communication.

Martin Vincent is a member of the Animal Health Service of the Food and Agriculture Organization of the United Nations. His responsibilities are in the area of early warning and response to disease emergencies. After obtaining his doctorate in veterinary medicine in 1993, he entered the French National School of Veterinary Services, where he studied veterinary public health and animal disease control and worked with various disease surveillance and disease control programs, including at the epidemiology unit of the Central Veterinary Laboratory in Zimbabwe.

Lin-Fa Wang is Senior Principal Research Scientist at the Australian Animal Health Laboratory, Geelong. He is also a project leader of the Australian Biosecurity Cooperative Research Centre for Emerging Infectious Diseases in Brisbane. His research interests include identification and characterization of new and emerging infectious agents, development of multiplex diagnostic tests, the study of virus-host interactions, and the characterization of antigen-antibody bindings.

Index

The letter *t* following a page number indicates a table.

A

absorptive capacity, and animal waste, 39–40
access to products, for poor people, 16
adventure travel, 127–28
affordability of products, for poor people, 16
Africa, rinderpest in, 65–66
African swine fever, 161. *See also* disease(s)
agribusiness: enterprise costs and, 21–22; pork and, 17–19. *See also* economics
agriculture: avian influenza and, 108–10; dry land and, 14; Green Revolution in, 19; history of, 43–46; overview of population and, 11–13; purpose of, 12; rain forests and, 14; supply chain history and, 52–53; variable control in, 22; water use and, 36; zoonoses and, 122, 123–25
agroterrorism, 49
Alliance for Prudent Use of Antibiotics (APUA), 93
American Association of Swine Veterinarians (AASV), 16, 17*t*
Animal and Plant Health Inspection Service (APHIS), 63
animal domestication, 44, 52

Animal Health Institute, 49, 93
animal-human contact, increase in, 37
Animal Plagues (Flemming), 62, 63, 64
animal welfare, 51–60. *See also* husbandry
antibiotics: resistance to, 92, 96–97; used for animals, 92–93, 94–95*t*, 95–96
antimicrobials, 47–48, 63–64
aquaculture: avian influenza and, 110; environment and, 86–87; increase in, 84–85; offshore, 85–90; research and development in, 88–89; United States and, 84–85
aquatic birds, 102, 103
Aravan virus, 146
Asia: AASV membership in, 17*t*; livestock demand in, 33; livestock production in, 35; milk consumption in, 33; percentage of total human population, 17*t*; poultry in, 109–10, 111
availability of products, for poor people, 16
avian influenza, 2; classification of, 104–6; compartmentalization of, 103; control of, 115–16; cultural practices and, 113–14; in ducks, 1 05; ecological barriers and, 115; economics and, 68; emergence of, 107–8; farming systems and, 108–11; fish farms and, 110; globalization and, 37, 77; host range, 106–7; live poultry markets and, 111–12;